Nelson Gaspar Dip Júnior

MicroRNA Expression Analysis in Urothelial Bladder Carcinoma

Nelson Gaspar Dip Júnior

MicroRNA Expression Analysis in Urothelial Bladder Carcinoma

Epigenetics in the carcinogenesis of Bladder Cancer

ScienciaScripts

Imprint

Cover image: www.ingimage.com

This book is a translation from the original published under ISBN 978-3-330-77194-9.

Publisher:
Sciencia Scripts
is a trademark of
Dodo Books Indian Ocean Ltd. and OmniScriptum S.R.L publishing group

120 High Road, East Finchley, London, N2 9ED, United Kingdom
Str. Armeneasca 28/1, office 1, Chisinau MD-2012, Republic of Moldova, Europe
Managing Directors: Ieva Konstantinova, Victoria Ursu
info@omniscriptum.com

Printed at: see last page
ISBN: 978-620-8-64041-5

CONTENTS

Thanks

To God in the first place, because without Him none of this would be possible.

To Prof. Dr. Kàtia, my advisor, for having welcomed me with open arms and heart, for her affection and understanding and for her maternal patience in teaching each one of us with rigor and dedication. It's people like you who make a better world. Thank you very much for your unforgettable time in my life.

To my great "sister" Sabrina Thalita dos Reis, for her friendship and patience, for her daring to grow more and more, for teaching me the best ways on this difficult journey. Sà, there are no words here to express how important you are in my life! Thank you so much!

To Prof. Dr. Miguel Srougi, head of the Urology department, for his immense spirit of leadership, simplicity and appreciation of the human being. Thank you very much for accepting me into this postgraduate program and for showing me that it is always possible to go one step further.

To Prof. Dr. Marcos Francisco DallOglio, head of Uro-oncology, for his example of competence and determination, and for supporting my training and professional growth.

To Dr. Carlos Alberto Lenzi, for his constant encouragement of my success, for his simple way of being, for having welcomed me like a son. Without you, everything would be much more difficult. Thank you!

Daniel Abe and Endric Hasegawa, friends of all hours, on whom I could count in every moment of joy and difficulty. I am eternally grateful for everything they taught me and for making me a better person every day.

To my eternal friend Rodrigo Alessandro Parreira, for the direct partnership, the friendly shoulder and the unceasing strength he always gave me. I can't thank you enough!

To Prof. Dr. Homero, coordinator of the Postgraduate Committee of the

Urology Discipline at USP, for the seriousness with which he conducts this program and for always being accessible to solve all my difficulties.

To the doctors and friends of the LIM-55 Medical Research Laboratory, José Pontes Junior, Alberto Azoubel Antunes, Iran, Camila, Nayara, Caio, Denis, Luciana, Manuel, Michele and Clàudia, for all the help and affection they gave me. Please know that without you, this learning experience would not have been possible.

To the secretaries of the Urology department, Elisa, Tereza and Iones, for their attention, time and promptness in always helping me.

Finally, I would like to thank the members of the Urology department at HCFMUSP: doctors, postgraduate students, residents and staff for their support.

I dedicate this work to my mother Luiza and my siblings Luis Fernando and Ana Cristina for their tireless strength and constant encouragement for my personal and professional growth.

1 INTRODUCTION

1.1 General considerations

Bladder cancer (BC) is the second most common urological malignant tumor and one of the most studied neoplasms today, with a history and biology that are still not well defined. Its development is related to environmental exposures which, through genetic and epigenetic mechanisms, alter the cellular machinery, leading to the installation of the carcinogenic process. Worldwide, it is responsible for approximately 386,000 new cases and 150,000 deaths a year (Jemal et al., 2011), and is considered a pathology with a major socio-economic impact and extremely high costs for health systems (Botteman et al., 2003).

Conventional clinical and pathological parameters are used to grade and stage this neoplasm and are the only tools currently used to predict the outcome of the disease. However, the predictive ability of these parameters is limited and there is a lack of data to allow a prospective analysis of the risks of progression and the behavior of CaB.

The concept that CaB is a multi-stage disease is supported by a range of scientific evidence and a range of alterations are required for the tumor to present clinically. As such, it has been used as one of the most important sources of information on mutational events that trigger carcinogenic pathways and the development of human solid tumors (Knowles, 2008; McConkey et al., 2010).

Although the genetic-molecular pathways have been relatively well demonstrated and some tumor markers have been established, there are many questions to be answered regarding the biological behavior of the disease, and new methods are needed to predict the behavior of CaB more specifically.

1.2 Epidemiology of Bladder Cancer

Cancer is one of the biggest public health problems in many parts of the world.

According to the *National Cancer Institute*, one in four deaths in the United States (US) is currently due to cancer, making it the second leading cause of death, accounting for 23.2% of all deaths in the country.

CaB is the second most common tumor of the genitourinary tract (Enokida and Nakagawa, 2008), ranking 7th among tumors and the 9th leading cause of death. In Brazil, 3002 deaths were recorded in 2009 (2090 men and 912 women) and the projection for 2012 is 8900 new cases (www.inca.gov.br). From birth to death, the chance of a man developing BC is 3.8% and a woman 1.2%, including the invasive type and carcinoma *in situ* (*Cis*).

It is a rare tumor before the age of 40, with a significant increase after the seventh decade of life (Jemal et al., 2011). Although the tumor is more frequent in men, there is evidence to show that it has a more aggressive behavior in women (Mungan et al., 2000). The higher incidence of these tumors in men is not completely explained by differences in smoking and occupational habits, the two main risk factors for the disease. When the incidence and mortality in women are taken into account, it seems that multiparous women have a lower risk than nulliparous women, probably due to the hormonal changes related to pregnancy, and this risk may become lower and lower with increasing parity (Cantor et al., 1992).

Biological variations can also modify the expression and action of genes related to the various phases of carcinogenesis, such as the conversion of pro-carcinogens into carcinogens, carcinogen detoxification and DNA repair.

Eighty-six percent of BCCs are diagnosed as localized, 8% with locorregional extension and 4% already as metastatic disease. Five-year survival has been increasing, with 74% in 1975-1977, 78% in 1984-1986 and 82% in 1999-2005, with an average mortality reduction of 5% between 1990 and 2006 (Jemal et al., 2011). The improvement in these rates is directly related to early diagnosis and the greater availability and effectiveness of treatment.

There is a significant impact on survival when the different tumor stages are taken into account. In the USA, six-year survival is 94% for *Cis*, 74% for pTa and pT1 tumors, 36% for locoregional disease and only 6% for disseminated CaB (Jemal et al., 2011).

1.2.1 Environmental risk factors

The most well-established risk factor for BCC is cigarette smoking, although this association is not as strong as that observed between smoking and the development of respiratory malignancies. Despite this, smoking increases the risk of tumors by two to four times, and increasing the intensity and/or duration of consumption is directly related to an increase in this risk, with an average latency period of 20 to 30 years, so that 30 to 50% of CaB are caused by cigarette use (Kirkali et al., 2005). Metabolic enzymes, vitamins and other agents can modify smoking-induced susceptibility, and the risk returns to baseline levels only after the individual has stopped smoking for 20 to 30 years.

Occupation is the second most important risk factor for the disease. It has been estimated that occupational exposure may be responsible for up to 20% of all bladder cancers. Exposure to β-naphthylamine, 4-aminobiphenyl (ABP) and benzidine, especially among workers in paint and rubber industries, show a direct relationship with the development of the disease. However, there are many other strong candidate carcinogens such as orthotoluidine, which is used in the manufacture of paints, rubber, pharmaceuticals and pesticides (Markowitz and Levin, 2004). In fact, many occupations have been linked to an increased risk of developing CaB, especially exposure to aromatic amines (arylamines) and also to aluminum, iron, coal and diesel (Theriault et al., 1984; Boffetta and Silverman, 2001; Gaertner and Theriault, 2002).

Chronic urinary infection is associated with the development of BAC, especially squamous cell carcinoma. This type of tumor can occur in patients who have suffered spinal cord trauma and in patients who have been probed for a long time, where repeated infections are common. The chronic inflammatory process can generate nitrites and nitrosamines, which lead to increased cell proliferation and genetic errors.

1.3 Bladder Cancer Management

Many characteristics of BAC have been studied in an attempt to predict the behavior of the tumor. Tumor staging and grading are fundamental for therapeutic decisions, and understanding the epidemiology and screening strategies can be useful in the prevention and early detection of the disease.

Although the diagnostic and therapeutic arsenal is very broad and every effort has been made to improve survival, CUB still suffers from unsatisfactory responses to treatment, disease progression and high mortality rates. This is due to its rapid progression and late diagnosis, the unpredictability of the lesions' behavior and the lack of methods to predict it. There is therefore an urgent need for other tools that will allow us to classify and predict the evolutionary pattern of CUB more reliably, especially molecular biology techniques using reliable and specific tumor markers.

1.3.1 Histological types

The most common histological type is urothelial carcinoma of the bladder (UCB), which occurs in 80 to 90% of cases and can present in a wide variety of ways , from a small, well-differentiated, non-invasive intravesical lesion to advanced disease that invades the bladder wall and adjacent organs, with the main prognostic factors being tumor grade and stage (McConkey et al., 2010).

Other types of tumor of epithelial origin are less common and include squamous cell carcinoma, related to chronic urinary infections and infestation by *Schistosoma hematobium*, and adenocarcinoma, which can be derived from the urachus or primary from the bladder (Heney, 1992). Mesenchymal and lymphoreticular tumors also affect the bladder, but are rare.

1.3.2 Tumor staging and grading

1.3.2.1 TNM staging

The pathological stage is one of the most important prognostic factors in CUB and is critical for decision-making and patient follow-up. The most commonly used system is that which evaluates tumor extension (T), lymph node involvement (N) and the presence of metastases (M), updated periodically by the American Board of Cancer (AJCC) (Table 1).

In simplified terms, staging discriminates between two main types of tumors with important implications for therapeutic decisions. CUB, wrongly called "superficial", can be classified as non-invasive (pTa) or invasive in the lamina propria (pT1), and invasive CUB is that which affects at least the muscularis propria or detrusor muscle, and is staged as pT2. Involvement of the perivesical fat classifies it as pT3 and invasion of adjacent organs and the pelvic wall as pT4. Between 70 and 80% of bladder tumors are pTa or pT1 and are characterized by high recurrence rates (50 to 70%), with only 10 to 15% progressing to a higher grade or stage. Those that are already invasive at diagnosis, which account for 10 to 20% of cases, tend to progress rapidly and have an unfavorable prognosis (Borden et al., 2005).

Despite this distinction between tumor types, it is still very difficult to absolutely differentiate which tumors will progress and/or recur after initial treatment, as tumors of similar morphology can behave differently. This is relevant at a time when therapeutic modalities, both curative and palliative, have significant degrees of morbidity.

Table 1 - TNM/AJCC 2010 classification

Primary Tumor (T)	
Tx	Primary tumor cannot be assessed
T0	No evidence of primary tumor
Ta	Non-invasive papillary tumor

Tis		Carcinoma *in situ* (*Cis*)
T1		Invade your own blade
T2	T2a	Invades own muscle superficially
	T2b	Invades his own muscle deeply
T3	T3a	Invades perivesical fat microscopically
	T3b	Invades the perivesical fat macroscopically
T4	T4a	Invades the prostatic stroma, uterus or vagina
	T4b	Invades the pelvic or abdominal wall
Lymph nodes (N)		
Nx		Lymph nodes cannot be assessed
N0		No evidence of lymph node metastasis
N1		Single positive lymph node in primary drainage region
N2		Multiple lymph nodes in primary drainage areas
N3		Positive common iliac chain
Distant metastases (M)		
Mx		Metastases cannot be assessed
M0		No evidence of distant metastasis
M1		Presence of distant metastases

1.3.2.2 Histological grading

Histological grade is, along with stage, the most important risk factor for the progression of neoplastic lesions in CUB. The system currently adopted is that published by the WHO/ISUP.

- Flat lesions

o Flat lesions with atypia

o Carcinoma *in situ* (*Cis*)

- Papillary lesions o Papilloma o Urothelial neoplasm with low malignant potential (UNMP)

○ Low-grade papillary carcinoma ○ High-grade papillary carcinoma

In an attempt to simplify the language and understanding between pathologists, urologists and oncologists, the WHO/ISUP system has renamed papillary urothelial carcinomas into just two categories: low-grade and high-grade. Low-grade papillary urothelial carcinoma has a general appearance with minimal variations in architecture and/or cytological characteristics, which are easily recognized. High-grade tumours are characterized by a disorganized appearance based on significant architectural and cytological abnormalities. Several studies have validated the applicability of this grading system. Desai et al. (2000) studied 120 patients with pTa and pT1 tumors using the WHO/ISUP classification system and their relationship with immunohistochemical patterns and observed the following in Table 2. Although papillomas do not show recurrence or progression and NUBPM only recurrence, low and high-grade lesions showed progression and, in some cases, resulted in death.

Table 2 - Prognosis of urothelial neoplasms according to Desai et al., 2000

	Papilloma	NUBPM	Low grade	High degree
Recurrence	0	33,3%	64,1%	56,4%
Progress	0	0	10,5%	27,1%
Invasion of your own blade	0	0	2,6%	8,3%
Detrusor invasion	0	0	5,3%	6,3%
Metastases	0	0	10,6%	25%

1.3.3 Diagnostic methods

Various tools have helped in the prevention and diagnosis of CUB, but they are still somewhat unspecific when some aspects are considered.

Screening aims to improve survival by detecting tumors early. Computational methods suggest that it can be advantageous and reduce mortality in high-risk individuals. However, its role has not yet been fully established (Kirkali et al.,

2005).

The most common symptom is painless hematuria, which occurs in approximately 85% of patients (Kirkali et al., 2005). The vast majority of patients are diagnosed through this typical sign of suspicion, associated with urinary cytology and cystoscopy, methods which make the cost of following up the disease extremely high (Babjuk et al., 2009).

Computed Tomography (CT) and Magnetic Resonance Imaging (MRI) represent the main imaging methods for staging the disease. However, despite being high-tech methods, they are unable to differentiate between pT1 and pT3 lesions because they cannot identify the microscopic extent of CUB (Paik et al., 2000). Thus, the biggest problems with these methods are over- and under-staging errors (Tritschler et al., 2011). To improve this accuracy, interesting techniques such as positron emission tomography (PET-CT) and MRI with iron nanoparticles have recently been introduced (Eisner and Feldman, 2009; Belakhlef et al., 2012).

Transurethral resection (TUR) of bladder tumors provides diagnostic information and therapeutic benefits. The main objectives of TUR are to remove all tumor tissue if technically feasible, and to obtain good quality material that allows adequate histopathological analysis (Babjuk et al., 2009; Miyamoto and Epstein, 2010).

Molecular markers offer the potential to characterize urothelial neoplasms individually and more completely than histological evaluation alone. They can be used in the assessment of tumor recurrence, molecular staging, detection of advanced disease, identification of therapeutic targets, prediction of response to treatments and, above all, in the early detection of the disease even before its onset (Proctor et al., 2010). The growing advances in the molecular biology of urothelial bladder tumors have helped researchers to draw a direct link between genetic-molecular findings and clinical outcomes.

1.3.4 Treatment

The treatment of CaB depends mainly on its histological type, stage and grade (Miyamoto and Epstein, 2010).

Non-muscle-invasive neoplasms (pTa and pT1) frequently recur and progress to muscle-invasive disease in a limited number of cases, and are generally subject to more conservative treatment. RTU is always the first form of treatment for these neoplasms, followed by intravesical immunotherapy or chemotherapy. The treatment of choice for non-invasive CUB is immunotherapy based on the bacillus Calmette-Guérin (BCG), which does not yet have a standard protocol for use, in terms of the time and frequency of applications (Babjuk et al., 2009). Meta-analysis studies confirm the benefit of BCG after RTU, compared to RTU alone or associated with QT, in preventing recurrence and progression of non-invasive tumors. Maintenance therapy is always indicated for high-risk tumors. The ideal regimen has not yet been defined, but one of the most widely used empirical regimens is that of the *Southwest Oncology Group* (SWOG). Radical cystectomy is recommended in patients who have failed BCG. Delaying radical surgical treatment can lead to compromised cancer-specific survival (Fritsche et al., 2010).

In muscle-invasive tumors, cystectomy is the best way of controlling the disease and provides the highest survival rates (Herr et al., 2004), and should be performed early due to the high rate of progression of these tumors. Gore et al. (2009) showed that the earlier it is performed, the higher the cancer-specific survival and the lower the mortality, and that when there is a delay of more than three months in radical surgical treatment, these parameters are reversed. The *National Comprehensive Cancer Network* (NCCN) protocol and many other protocols define radical cystectomy associated with pelvic lymphadenectomy as the gold standard of therapy for muscle-invasive BC, while alternative treatments are reserved for cases where there are severe comorbidities (Montie et al., 2009; Gore et al., 2009). Finally, bladder preservation protocols can be applied to selected patients. These protocols have not yet been defined and various forms of treatment are applied and/or combined with each other, and include radical TURP, intravesical QT, radiotherapy, intravesical brachytherapy, partial cystectomy, among others.

1.4 Molecular Biology of Bladder Cancer

A large number of genetic events are involved in the etiology, progression and response to treatment of CUB (Garcia del Muro et al., 2004). Elucidating the molecular pathways involved in the carcinogenic process of the disease is essential for understanding its etiopathogenesis and behavior.

1.4.1 Genetic changes in non-invasive CUB

The carcinogenic pathways from which low-grade non-invasive papillary tumors and high-grade, invasive carcinomas derive are specific and mutually exclusive and are illustrated in Figure 1 (van Rhijn et al., 2004; Bakkar et al., 2003; Pandith et al., 2010). Most bladder malignancies are non-muscle-invasive in their initial presentation and their main carcinogenic route is via a mutation in the gene encoding the fibroblast growth factor receptor type 3 (FGFR3). However, less commonly, mutations in the RAS gene have also been described.

The FGFR3 gene, located in chromosome region 4p16.3 (Thompson et al., 1991) has 18 exons and belongs to the family of tyrosine kinase growth factor receptors, involved in functions related to embryogenesis and maintenance of tissue homeostasis (Pandith et al., 2010). These receptors regulate various biological processes, including cell proliferation, differentiation and migration, as well as apoptosis (Ornitz et al., 1996). They have a common structure comprising an extracellular domain, a hydrophobic transmembrane domain and an intracellular tyrosine kinase domain. The binding of FGF to its receptor FGFR3 leads to the stimulation of second messengers via the intracellular domain. This activation pathway can produce well-differentiated, low-grade tumors. Mutations or other alterations that lead to FGFR3 overactivity alter cell proliferation, but have little effect on differentiation and apoptosis, providing an advantage for cancer cell growth while maintaining their genomic stability.

Two mechanisms are capable of leading to the abnormal activity of FGFR3, i.e. the t(4;14) translocation which results in overexpression of the protein, and the punctiform mutation which results in anomalous activation of the receptor without the need for the ligand. The first evidence that FGFR3 could be an oncogene was observed in multiple myeloma, a plasma cell neoplasm, where altered expression of the gene was observed in 10 to 25% of patients. FGFR3 mutations in CUB were first reported by Cappellen et al. (1999), who identified them in 35% of these tumors. Mutations in codons 248, 249 and 375 comprise more than 95% of all FGFR3 mutations, with codon 249 being responsible for approximately 70% of them.

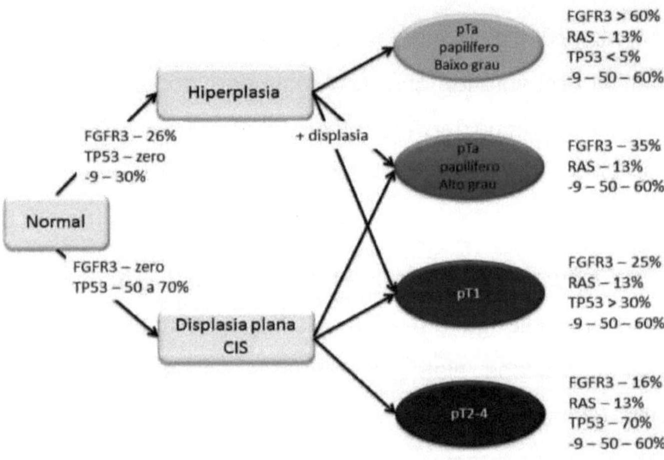

Figure 1 - Pathways of carcinogenesis in urothelial carcinoma of the bladder

The most frequent FGFR3 mutations can be caused by smoking or environmental exposure to carcinogens which create an extracellular cysteine residue and activate the tyrosine kinase domain, leading to a decrease in specificity for the ligand and consequent dimerization and autophosphorylation of the intracellular domain. van Rhijn et al. (2001) reported an association between the FGFR3 mutation and the presence of low-grade urothelial carcinomas or papillomas in more than 70% of cases of pTa tumors. In muscle-invasive tumors, these mutations may be present, but at very low rates (up to 15% of cases). Although these literature data point to mutated FGFR3 as a molecular marker of pTa, they are controversial in predicting the risk of recurrence and progression of the disease (Pandith et al., 2010).

In 2007, Tomlinson et al. designed a study to investigate the mutation in the FGFR3 gene and its association with the overexpression of its protein product, correlating them with tumor stage and grade, and 85% of the tumors that showed the mutation also had protein overexpression of FGFR3. It seems possible that mutations in FGFR3 are an early event in the development of this type of tumor and, in most cases, may protect against progression to muscle-invasive disease.

Mutations in the RAS oncogene have also been linked to non-invasive tumors. In 1982, Der et al. discovered that the HRAS gene, one of the first human oncogenes described, was also associated with CUB and was identified in the T24 cell line. There are three genes in the RAS family, H-RAS, K-RAS and N-RAS, which are directly involved in the development of 30% of human cancers (van der Weyden and Adams, 2007). RAS acts by regulating and controlling various cellular functions such as proliferation, differentiation, motility and apoptosis, in response to extracellular signals. In CUB, it seems to act through the activation of the MAPK (mitogen-activated protein kinase) pathway or the AKT/STAT pathways (Jebar et al., 2005). Mo et al. (2007) studied H-RAS and the behavior of non-invasive bladder tumors and demonstrated a relationship between the oncogene and tumor grade and aggressiveness. The authors concluded that overactivation of H-RAS by punctiform mutation and overexpression is necessary and sufficient to induce non-invasive bladder tumors and that inhibition of this activity could be a therapeutic alternative. Finally, Przybojewska et al. (2000) showed that H-RAS is active in 84% of non-invasive CUB specimens. Mutations in the N-RAS gene were similar to those in H-RAS, suggesting a relationship between them in bladder neoplasia, while alterations in K-RAS appear to be a rare event.

Interestingly, RAS and FGFR3 gene mutations do not seem to occur concomitantly and are therefore mutually exclusive events, indicating the biological equivalence of these two types of mutation (Jebar et al., 2005).

Since the activation of FGFR3 through mutation is the key event in the development of low-grade pTa tumors, its role as the first molecular marker of non-aggressive disease is speculated (Rieger-Christ et al., 2003). Furthermore, FGFR3 can be targeted by drugs and blocking the receptor with antibodies is of great interest, being considered as a potential therapeutic target in CUB. Martinez-Torrecuadrada et al. (2005) conducted a study to investigate the effect of the human single-chain Fv antibody (scFv) as a specific inhibitor of FGFR3 function. The authors report that they were able to block cell proliferation in the AcB RT112 tumor cell line, which expresses high levels of FGFR3.

1.4.2 Genetic changes in invasive CUB

Most of the known genetic events in CUB are described in invasive tumors and many of them, such as the p53 gene mutation, retinoblastoma (RB1) and PTEN, are associated with poor prognosis. Invasive urothelial carcinomas of the bladder are more aggressive neoplasms with high genetic instability (Knowles, 2008).

The p53 gene product is a tumor suppressor protein that responds to various cellular stress signals by regulating the transcription of a series of genes that induce cell cycle arrest, apoptosis, senescence, DNA repair and alterations in cell metabolism. Somatic mutations of p53 are described in more than half of human neoplasms and germline mutations are involved in hereditary syndromes that promote the development of a series of tumors. Unlike FGFR3, loss of function of the p53 gene leads to genomic instability that is important in the generation of high-grade and high-stage tumors (Hainaut and Hollstein, 2000). Esrig et al. (1994) and Sarkis et al. (1994) were the first to demonstrate that p53 alterations are important markers of recurrence and mortality in CUB. The p21 gene, also known as CDKN1A, encodes an inhibitor of cyclins CDK2 and CDK4, functioning as a regulator of the cell cycle. The expression of this gene is controlled by the p53 protein, exerting a negative effect on the G1 phase of the cell cycle in the face of a variety of stresses. Joint abnormalities of p21 and p53 predict poor prognosis and shorter disease-free survival.

The susceptibility of the RB1 gene, a prototype tumor suppressor gene, has been associated with the development and/or progression of CUB. This phosphoprotein is a negative regulator of the cell cycle and stabilizes heterochromatin, maintaining its structure. Mutations in this gene are markedly associated with the development of childhood retinoblastoma, osteogenic sarcoma and bladder cancer (www.ncbi.nlm.nih.gov/gene). The inactivation of RB1 is linked to CUB, more specifically to invasive disease with worse behavior, speculating its possible use as a prognostic marker. Evaluating the role of RB1 in bladder tumors, Gallucci et al. in 2005 observed that its heterozygous deletion was associated with advanced stages of the disease (pT3-pT4). The authors concluded with the finding that 86% of the tumors had a heterozygous deletion and 11% a homozygous deletion of the RB1 gene, and this behavior was associated with higher grades, advanced stages and reduced survival. Cordon-Cardo et al. (1992) evaluated 48 tumors from radical cystectomy and showed that of the 38 patients with muscle-invasive disease, 34% had altered RB1 expression, while this mutation was practically absent in non-invasive tumors. They concluded that tumors with these mutations have more aggressive behavior and shorter survival.

Since more than half of invasive tumors have deficiencies in the p53 and/or RB1 pathways, restoring the functions of these pathways could resume cellular physiological processes, promote apoptosis, prevent progression and control tumor growth (Wu, 2009). Several recently discovered small molecules with the ability to bind to the mutated p53 gene or truncated protein are capable of restoring their functions. Two prototypes are CP-31398 and PRIMA-1, capable of reactivating p53 function and inducing massive apoptosis.

The phosphatase and tensin homolog (PTEN) gene is located on the long arm of chromosome 10 (10q23) and also functions as a traditional tumor suppressor, with roles in controlling cell proliferation, migration and invasion through the PI3K/AKT/mTOR pathway (Wu, 2009; McConckey et al., 2010). Despite having an influence on the development of non-invasive bladder tumors, PTEN is much more associated with the promoter and progression pathways of invasive CUB. Although there is evidence to suggest its role in neoplastic initiation and progression, it seems that PTEN is not able to promote them on its own (Tsuruta et al., 2006). Recent data show that when PTEN loss of function is associated with p53 mutations, the invasive tumor sets in and progresses more rapidly, with a worse prognosis and shorter survival (Puzio-Kuter et al., 2009).

Associations of genetic alterations within the carcinogenic pathway of invasive CUB appear to be the main event leading to the initiation and progression of these urothelial tumors (Figure 1).

1.4.3 Epigenetics of CUB

Genetic alterations alone cannot explain the molecular diversity of cancer, and other mechanisms can also affect gene expression and signaling pathways. Epigenetic changes such as DNA hypermethylation and histone deacetylation, which occur without modifying the DNA structure, appear to contribute to malignant transformation and CUB progression (Dalmay, 2008; Enokida and Nakagawa, 2008) and can be promoted by exposure to external stimuli, including smoking, diet and carcinogens.

A variety of genes important in various cellular processes can show DNA hypermethylation at rates ranging from 1% to 98% (Kim et al., 2005; Friedrich et al., 2005; Marsit et al., 2007; Yates et al., 2007; Ellinger et al., 2008; Lodygin et al., 2008). In addition, some of these epigenetic changes can be regulated by microRNA. Hypermethylation can be detected in the normal urothelium and in the *Cis* of patients with invasive tumors, indicating that these epigenetic aberrations are already present at early stages of the disease (Brait et al., 2008). Considering the current model of bladder carcinogenesis, it has been suggested that hypermethylation of genes is more typical of invasive tumors and has been related to worse prognosis and lower survival, so these alterations have been suggested as biomarkers for CUB. Brait et al. (2008), using a group of seven genes, demonstrated that the methylation of their promoter areas allows invasive and non-invasive disease to be stratified. Finally, Yates et al. (2007) reported that hypermethylation of the E-cadherin promoter area was associated with disease progression and cancer death.

Another epigenetic mechanism is the repression of transcription through the interaction of microRNA (miRNA) with specific messenger RNA (mRNA) sequences, which will be discussed below.

1.4.4 Micro RNA

After their discovery almost 20 years ago (Lee et al., 1993), miRNAs have been recognized as molecules that act specifically in the post-transcriptional control of the majority of the eukaryotic genome. They are a family of small RNAs ranging from 19 to 25 nucleotides expressed in a wide variety of organisms, encompassing plants, worms and mammals including man (Pillai et al., 2005). Many miRNAs are highly conserved between species and their processing machinery can be found in archaea and eubacteria, proving their ancestral character. Currently, there are more than 1400 miRNA, related to the regulation of more than 30% of human genes (www.mirnabodymap.org; Lewis et al.,

2005) involved in multiple processes of cell development and differentiation, apoptosis, homeostasis and metabolic pathways (Ambros, 2003; Bartel, 2004; Blenkiron and Miska, 2007).

1.4.4.1 Biogenesis of miRNA

After its transcription by RNA polymerase II, the primary precursor of miRNA, called pri-miRNA, is subjected to the action of the nuclear microprocessor complex Drosha and then converted into pre-miRNA, a double-stranded molecule of approximately 60-70 nucleotides (Han et al., 2004; Lee et al., 2004; Gregory et al., 2004; Kim, 2005). The pre-miRNA is exported from the nucleus to the cytoplasm by Exportin-5, a protein specialized in the nucleocytoplasmic transport of macromolecules, including ribonucleic acids (Yi et al., 2003). Once in the cytoplasm, the pre-miRNA is cleaved by the Dicer enzyme, transforming it into a small (19 to 25 nucleotides) double-stranded miRNA, known as a duplex miRNA. This, in turn, is again affected by Dicer, which cleaves the double strand and produces the mature single-stranded miRNA, which is then incorporated into an effector complex called RISC (RNA-induced silencing complex) (Lee et al., 2003; Carmell and Hannon, 2004; Bartel, 2004). The RISC guides the mature miRNA to its target mRNA, where a perfect or incomplete base complementarity interaction will occur, leading to the cleavage of the mRNA or the inhibition of protein translation, respectively (Meister et al., 2004; Pillai, 2005). Figure 2 summarizes all these processes.

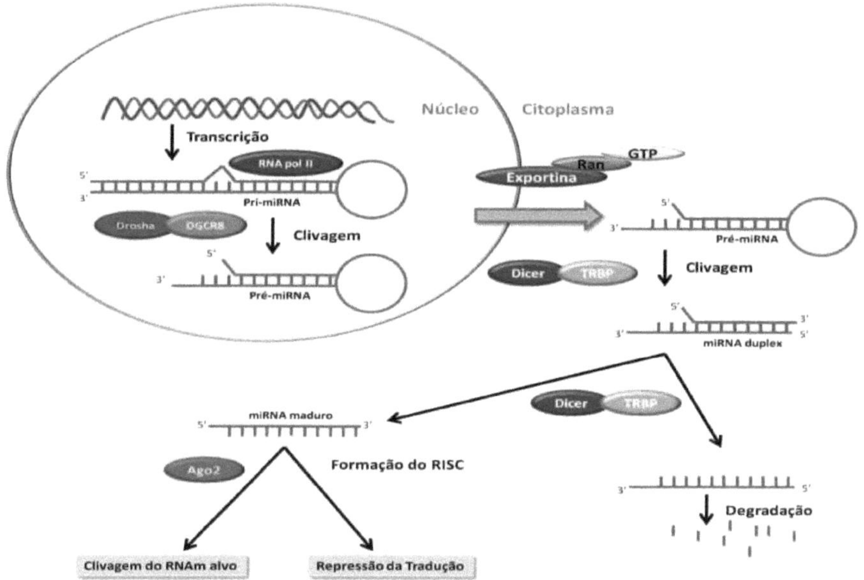

Figure 2 - Schematic showing miRNA biogenesis

1.4.4.2 MicroRNA functions

Although the vast majority of studies have focused on the role of miRNAs in the development and progression of diseases, diagnosis, prognosis and therapeutic strategies, they are fundamental in the phenomena of embryogenesis, cell development and differentiation, proliferation and metabolism (Dalmay, 2008).

Within cancer research, miRNAs have been shown to be tumor suppressors or oncogenes, demonstrating alterations that can characterize different types of cancer (Calin and Croce, 2006; Blenkiron and Miska, 2007). Although there are studies exploring miRNA expression profiles in CUB, the data is still scarce and the field of exploration quite vast (Gottardo et al., 2007; Gregory et al., 2008; Neely et al., 2008; Ichimi et al., 2009; Veerla et al., 2009).

2. Objectives

The objectives of this study are:

1.5 Primary

- Characterizing a microRNA expression profile in urothelial bladder carcinoma

1.6 Secondary

- To compare the expression pattern of the miRNAs studied in two different tumor groups, i.e. invasive high-grade urothelial carcinoma and non-invasive low-grade urothelial carcinoma.
- Relating the microRNA expression profile to recurrence and progression of the neoplasm in patients surgically treated for CUB

3. METHODS

1.7 Patients

The expression profile of 14 miRNAs from 65 patients divided into three groups was studied: 30 patients with low-grade non-muscle-invasive CUB (pTa) who underwent transurethral resection, 30 patients with high-grade muscle-invasive CUB (pT2-3) who underwent radical cystectomy and five control patients with a normal bladder without cancer who underwent open surgical treatment for benign prostatic hyperplasia, between January 2008 and December 2009, at the Hospital das Clinicas da Faculdade de Medicina da Universidade de Sâo Paulo (HCFMUSP) and Instituto do Câncer do Estado de Sâo Paulo (ICESP) by Prof. Dr. Miguel Srougi's team. Dr. Miguel Srougi. Considering the three groups studied, 72.3% were male, with an overall mean and median age of 66 years, ranging from 41 to 82 years. Table 3 shows the demographic characteristics of the three groups in more detail, with no statistical differences in age group between them (p = 0.29).

Table 3 - Demographic characteristics of the groups studied

	Low-grade non-invasive pTa (n = 30)			High invasive grade pT2-3 (n = 30)			Controls (n = 5)		
	Sex (%)	**Age (years)**		*Sex (%)*	**Age (years)**		*Sex (%)*	**Age (years)**	
		Average	Median (min-max)		Average	Median (min-max)		Average	Median (min-max)
Male	86,7	68,2	67,5 (47-82)	53,3	64,4	66 (41-79)	100	66	66 (61-71)
Female	13,3	61,8	61 (57-68)	46,7	65	67,5 (46-81)	0	-	-

The patients were informed about the objectives of this study and signed an informed consent form (Appendix B). The average follow-up time was 17.7 months, with a median of 16 months, ranging from

3 a 46. For pTa tumors, follow-up was done by cystoscopy and urinary cytology

every three months for the first 24 months, followed by the same tests every six months from the third to the fifth year after diagnosis. For invasive pT2-3 tumors, follow-up was done by quarterly abdominal and chest CT scans in the first two years, every six months from the third to the fifth year and annually from the fifth postoperative year onwards. Therapeutic interventions were carried out according to the needs of each case. This study was approved by the Ethics Committee of this institution under number 0176/10 (Annex A).

1.8 Macro and microscopic examination

The surgical specimens were examined fresh by the pathologist and the researcher who carried out this work, immediately after their resection, and a 1 cm fragment was sectioned[2], stored immediately in a 1.5 ml *Eppendorf* cryotube with 1 ml of RNA *holder*® (RNA fixative) and kept in a -80 °C freezer at the Urological Medical Research Laboratory (LIM-55) of the University of São Paulo Medical School (FMUSP).

After sectioning the fragment for miRNA extraction, the surgical specimens were fixed in 10% formalin for up to 24 hours. All specimens that had been submitted for RTU or radical cystectomy were histologically analyzed for the classic prognostic factors. The specimens were usually processed and embedded in paraffin, sectioned into 4 to 6 µm sections, stained with hematoxylin-eosin and analyzed under an optical microscope by the same pathologist, ensuring the presence of neoplasia in at least 75% of the sample. The following prognostic parameters were assessed:

a. Histological grading according to the WHO/ISUP 2004 classification.

b. TNM pathologic staging according to AJCC 2010.

1.9 RNA processing

1.9.1 Isolation of miRNA

The miRNA were isolated using the *mirVana* kit® (Ambion) according to the manufacturer's recommendations (Appendix C). This kit allows the isolation of all types of RNA. The specimens frozen at -80 °C were macerated and placed in a sterile 1.5 ml microcentrifuge tube. 500 µl of lysis buffer and 50 µl of homogenizing additive were then added to the tube and the solution left on ice for 10 minutes. Then 500 µl of phenol-chloroform acid was added and the samples were vortexed and centrifuged at a maximum speed of 10,000 rpm for 5 minutes at room temperature. The aqueous phase was removed to a new tube and a third of the volume of 100% ethanol was added, then the solution was transferred to a filter and centrifuged at 10,000 rpm for 15 seconds. The filter containing the total RNA was stored. Two thirds of 100% ethanol was added to the filtrate containing the miRNA. The solution was transferred to a new column and centrifuged at 10,000 rpm for 15 seconds. The samples were then washed with 700 µl of *wash solution 1/3* and centrifuged for 15 seconds at 10,000 rpm, followed by two more washes with 500 µl of *wash solution 2/3*, centrifuged at intervals for 15 seconds at 10,000 rpm. At this point, 100 µl of RNAse-free water at 95 °C was added to the filter and the samples centrifuged again at 10,000g for 15 seconds. The filtrate containing the miRNA was then stored in a -80 °C freezer until use. Concentration and purity were estimated using a Nanodrop® spectrophotometer (ND-1000, Wilmington, USA) (260/280 nM).

1.9.2 Synthesis of cDNA

Briefly, the miRNA was diluted in nuclease-free water and 3 µl of it was used, to which 0.15 µl of the dNTP mix (100 mM total), 0.19 µl of RNAse inhibitor (20 U/pl), 1,5 µl of enzyme buffer (RT Buffer 10X), 0.5 µl of *Multiscribe* ™ *RT enzyme* (50 U/µl), 3.66 µl of free water of nucleases and 1 µl of specific *primers* for each miRNA, totaling 10 µl. The mixtures were subjected to 16 °C for 30 minutes, 42 °C for 30 minutes and 85 °C for 5 minutes to synthesize the cDNA strand in a Veriti® thermal cycler (Applied Biosystems, California, USA).

Below is a schematic model of how miRNA complementary DNA is synthesized.

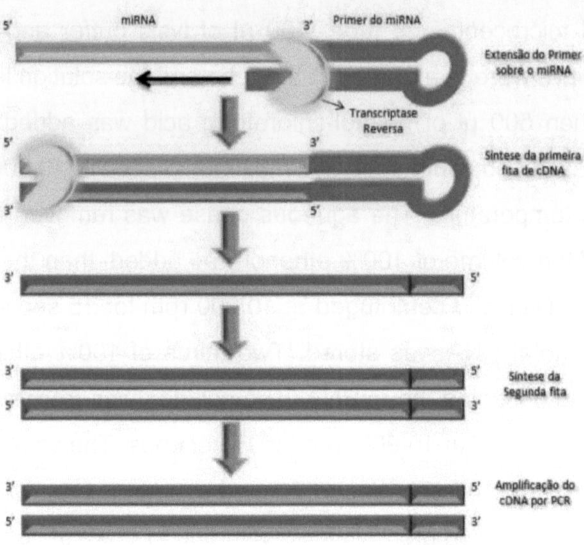

Figure 3 - Synthesis of complementary DNA

1.9.3 Amplification of miRNA

The *primers* used for miRNA amplification were purchased from Applied Biosystems, California, USA, which designs *primers* with the characteristics required for Real-Time PCR (RT-PCR) experiments on the *ABI 7500 Fast* thermal cycler.

The TaqMan® reagent (Applied Biosystems, California, USA) was used to quantify the samples. This protocol uses two fluorescent non primers and a double-labeled probe that anneals to the region between the primers. This double-labeling consists of a fluorophore that emits light when excited and a *quencher* that absorbs the light emitted by the fluorophore. During the PCR cycles, the probe is broken by the *Taq* polymerase in the extension step of the ring primer. This breakage of the probe eliminates absorption by the *quencher* of the emitted fluorescence, which can then be measured using a camera located on the top of the equipment. Quantifying the emission absorbed by the camera after the probe has broken allows the RT-PCR product to be detected (Figure 4). Briefly, the reaction was prepared by adding 5 µl of *MasterMix*, 3.5 µl of nuclease-free water, 1 µl of cDNA and 0.5 µl of the specific *primer* for each miRNA studied to PCR plates. Afterwards, the reactions were inserted into the qRT-PCR equipment and processed by the device for 2 minutes at 50 °C, 10 minutes at 95 °C and 40 thermal cycles of 15 seconds at 95 °C followed by 1 minute at 60 $^{(o)}$C. The expression values of each sample for each miRNA are shown in appendices D and E.

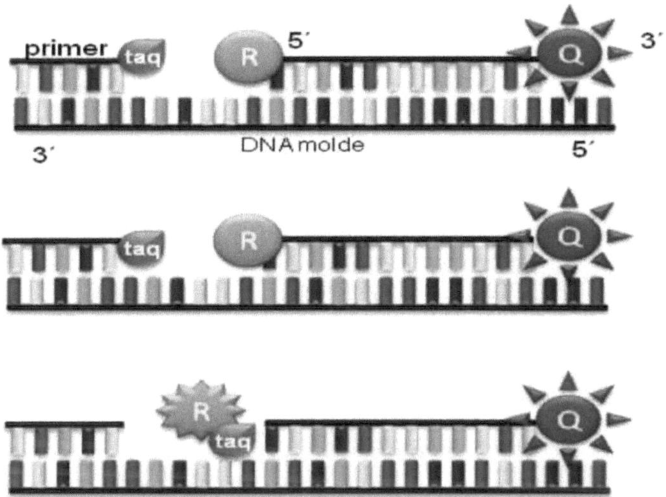

Figure 4 - Amplification of miRNA using the TaqMan® method

3.4 Analysis of results

The 14 miRNAs evaluated in this study, their characteristics and their possible target genes are shown in Tables 4 and 5. With the exception of miR-100, the choice of miRNAs for this study was based on data from the literature that demonstrated fundamental and/or promising roles for these miRNAs in the carcinogenic pathways of urothelial tumors. Specifically, miR-100 was selected for analysis because, in addition to being part of all the lines of research in our laboratory, there is scarce data on its action, both in the tumorigenic pathway of non-invasive and invasive neoplasia. The miRNA expression levels were obtained by relative quantification of the expression levels determined by the $2^{-\Delta\Delta(CT)}$) method, for which $\Delta\Delta CT = dCTi - dCT2$, where dCT_i = CT of the target miRNA, (tumor sample) - CT of the mean of the endogenous control (tumor sample), and dCT2 = CT of the mean of the controls (normal bladder tissue samples) - CT of the mean of the endogenous control (normal bladder tissue sample). In the logarithmic graph, this method standardizes the expression of the normal control as a baseline (represented by the number 1) and the relative expression of each miRNA for each tumor sample is shown in times the normal for more in cases of overexpression and less in cases of underexpression.

All reactions were carried out in duplicate and the small nucleolar RNA RNU43 and RNU48 (Applied Biosystems, CA, USA) used as endogenous controls. For expression analysis, in addition to the endogenous controls, we analyzed the expression levels of the same miRNA in normal, non-neoplastic bladder tissue as shown in the equation above.

Table 4 - MicroRNAs analyzed and their possible target genes

MicroRNA	Target gene	References
100	THAP2, SMARCA5, BAZ2A, FGFR3	Zhou et al., 2002; Bessière et al., 2008; Veerla et al., 2009; Catto et al., 2009
10a	FGFR3, HOXA-1	Veerla et al., 2009; Garzon et al., 2006
21	PTEN, p53	Neely et al., 2008; Wu et al., 2009; Catto et al., 2009; McConkey et al, 2010
205	p53, PTEN, ZEB-1, ZEB-2	Gottardo et al., 2007; Gregory et al., 2008; Neely et al., 2008
Let-7c	RAS, MYC	Reinhart et al., 2000; Johnson et al., 2005
125b	KRT-7, MUC-1, E2F3, p53	Ichimi et al., 2009; Le et al., 2009; Rajabi et al., 2010; Huang et al., 2011
143	RAS	Lin et al., 2009

145	KRT-7, FSCN-1, c- MYC/p53	Ichimi et al., 2009; Chiyomaru et al., 2010; Sachdeva et al., 2009
221	p27KIP1, DDIT4	Gottardo et al., 2007; Pineau et al., 2010
223	MEF2C, STMN-1	Gottardo et al., 2007; Wong et al., 2008
15a	BCL2	Calin et al., 2002
16-1	BCL2	Calin et al., 2002
199a	KRT7, mTOR, PODXL	Ichimi et al., 2009; Fornari et al., 2010; Cheung et al., 2011
452	Not yet defined	Veerla et al., 2009

Table 5 - Specifications of the microRNAs studied

MicroRNA	Chromosomal localization	Sequence	Number of Bases
100	11q24.1	AACUGUUUGCAGAGGAAACUGA	22
10a	17q21.32	UACCCUGUAGAUCCGAAUUUGUG	23
21	17q23.1	UAGCUUAUCAGACUGAUGUUGA	22
205	1q32.2	UCCUUCAUUCCACCGGAGUCUG	22
Let-7c	21q21.1	UGAGGUAGUAGGUUGUAUGGUU	22
125b	11q24.1	UCCCUGAGACCCUAACUUGUGA	22
143	5q32	UGAGAUGAAGCACUGUAGCUC	22
145	5q32	GUCCAGUUUUCCCAGGAAUCCCU	23
221	Xp11.3	AGCUACAUUGUCUGCUGGGUUUC	23
223	Xq12	UGUCAGUUUGUCAAAUACCCCA	22
15a	13q14.2	UAGCAGCACAUAAUGGUUUGUG	22
16-1	13q14.2	UAGCAGCACGUAAAUAUUGGCG	22
199a	19p13.2	CCCAGUGUUCAGACUACCUGUUC	23
452	Xq28	AACCCGUAGAUCCGAACUUGUG	22

Figure 5 shows the methodology applied and developed in this study in schematic form.

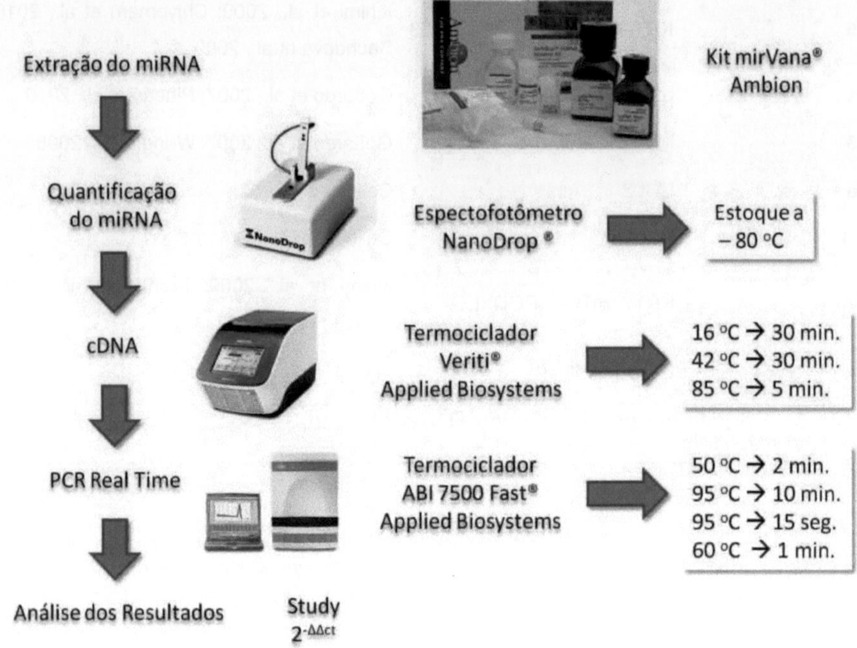

Figure 5 - Methodological scheme of the study

3.5 Statistical analysis

Statistical methods were used to compare the miRNA expression profile between the two groups of tumors and the prognostic factors. For homogeneous groups, we used the T-test to compare two groups and ANOVA for three or more groups. For non-homogeneous groups, we used the Mann-Whitney test to compare two groups and the Kruskal-Wallis test for three or more groups. The Chi-square test was used to compare groups on a nominal scale. The data was transformed into yogarithmic graphs for analysis and the expression of each sample for a given miRNA is relative to the control and expressed in times. The results were obtained using the statistical analysis program SPSS 19.0 for Windows and are presented as geometric means with a 95% confidence interval.

Kaplan-Meyer curves were also constructed to study relapse-free survival

(RFS) and cancer-specific survival (CSS), with the aim of relating the miRNA profiles to the behavior of CUB.

4. Results

4.1 General expression pattern in urothelial carcinoma of the bladder

The results of the expression of the 14 miRNAs in low-grade, non-invasive CUB and high-grade, invasive CUB are shown in Table 5 and Figures 6 and 7. Most of the miRNAs were underexpressed in the tumors analyzed, except for miR-100, 21 and 205 in pT2-3 tumors and miR- 10a in pTa tumors, which are overexpressed.

4.2 miRNA expression profile in low-grade carcinomas, pTa and high-grade carcinomas, pT2-3

miRNA 100, 10a, 21 and 205 showed differences in expression when comparing the two groups of tumors (Figures 6 and 7 and Table 6).

All low-grade pTa tumors showed under-expression of miR-100, while high-grade pT2-3 tumors showed over-expression in 57.7%. The average expression of miR-100 in low-grade pTa tumors was only 0.04 *versus* 24.39 in high-grade pT2-3 carcinomas ($p < 0.001$).

miR-10a showed an inverse expression profile in relation to miR-100, i.e. it was overexpressed in 73.3% of low-grade tumors, pTa, and underexpressed in 93.3% of high-grade tumors, pT2-3, with mean expressions of 46.38 and 0.23, respectively ($p < 0.001$).

miRNA 21 and 205 were also significantly overexpressed in high-grade pT2-3 tumors. The mean expression of miR-21 was 1.08 and 18.17 in low-grade, pTa and high-grade, pT2-3 tumors respectively ($p = 0.02$). The means of miR-205 in the same groups were 0.07 and 6.91 ($p < 0.001$).

Table 6 - Expression levels of the 14 miRNAs according to grade and stage

	Histological Grade Average Median (min-max)			**Pathological Staging** Mean Median (min-max)		
miRNA	*Low (n=30)*	*High (n=30)*	*p*	*pTa (n=30)*	*pT2/T3 (n=30)*	*p*
100	0,04 0,0008 (8,94^{-13}-0,44)	24,39 1,77 (0,02-526,6)	**< 0,001**	0,04 0,0008 (8,94^{-13}-0,44)	24,39 1,77 (0,02-526,6)	**< 0,001**
10a	46,38 4,88 (0,004-761,2)	0,23 0,06 (0,001-1,75)	**< 0,001**	46,38 4,88 (0,004-761,2)	0,23 0,06 (0,001-1,75)	**< 0,001**
21	1,08 0,4 (0,002-11,14)	18,17 0,65 (0,03-407,99)	**0,02**	1,08 0,4 (0,002-11,14)	18,17 0,65 (0,03-407,99)	**0,03**
205	0,07 0,04 (0,002-0,35)	6,91 0,65 (0,009-97,84)	**< 0,001**	0,07 0,04 (0,002-0,35)	6,91 0,65 (0,009-97,84)	**< 0,001**
Let7c	1,03 0,02 (6,3^{-5}-13,14)	0,29 0,1 (0,0003-1,41)	0,16	1,03 0,02 (6,3^{-5}-13,14)	0,29 0,1 (0,0003-1,41)	0,31
125b	0,15 0,08 (9,4^{-5}-0,76)	0,26 0,06 (0,0001-2,02)	0,92	0,15 0,08 (9,4^{-5}-0,76)	0,26 0,06 (0,0001-2,02)	0,99
143	0,18 0,009 (7,4^{-5}-4,13)	0,18 0,005 (1,7^{-6}-3,85)	0,99	0,18 0,009 (7,4^{-5}-4,13)	0,18 0,005 (1,7^{-6}-3,85)	0,76
145	1,61 0,2 (0,002-24,06)	0,66 0,13 (4,4^{-5}-10,25)	0,27	1,61 0,2 (0,002-24,06)	0,66 0,13 (4,4^{-5}-10,25)	0,48
221	1,22 0,3 (0,003-17,64)	0,48 0,34 (0,06-1,92)	0,89	1,22 0,3 (0,003-17,64)	0,48 0,34 (0,06-1,92)	0,98
223	0,49 0,1 (0,002-9,49)	1,007 0,29 (0,009-6,2)	0,21	0,49 0,1 (0,002-9,49)	1,007 0,29 (0,009-6,2)	0,41
15a	2,76 1,04 (0,1-15,3)	13,53 0,69 (0,02-331,1)	0,78	2,76 1,04 (0,1-15,3)	13,53 0,69 (0,02-331,1)	0,93
16-1	1,47 0,57 (2,6^{-5}-12,3)	0,76 0,54 (0,001-3,3)	0,81	1,47 0,57 (2,6^{-5}-12,3)	0,76 0,54 (0,001-3,3)	0,95
199a	0,36 0,13 (0,0008-2,7)	0,69 0,19 (0,002-6,78)	0,25	0,36 0,13 (0,0008-2,7)	0,69 0,19 (0,002-6,78)	0,52
452	1,42 0,03 (0,0001-39,87)	0,24 0,03 (0,001-3,69)	0,39	1,42 0,03 (0,0001-39,87)	0,24 0,03 (0,001-3,69)	0,68

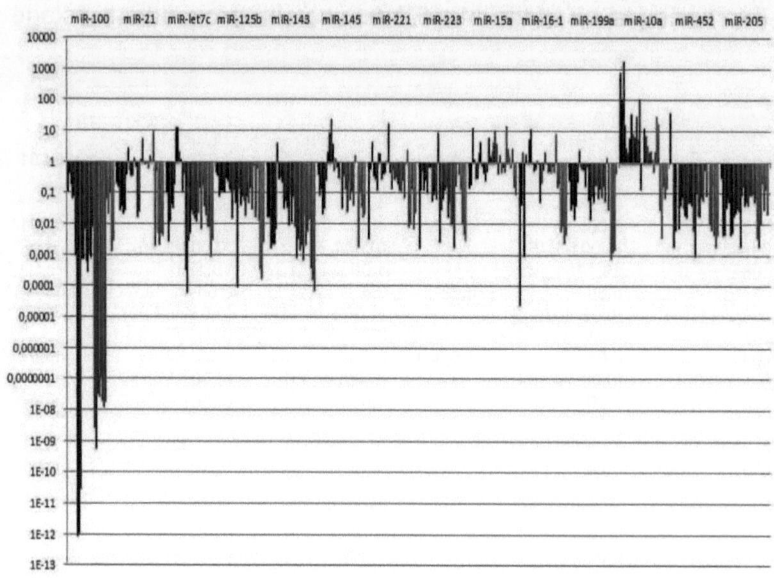

Figure 6 - Expression profile of the 14 miRNAs in low-grade pTa tumors

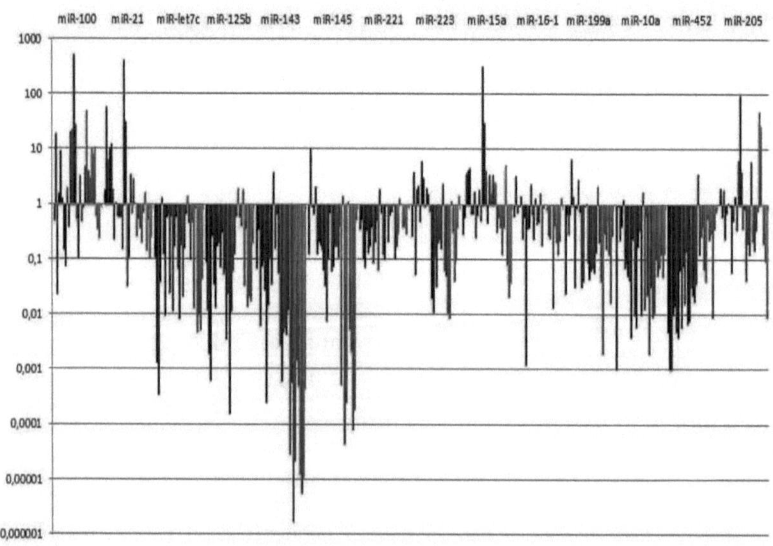

Figure 7 - Expression profile of the 14 miRNAs in high-grade pT2-3 tumors

4.3 miRNA expression profile, recurrence and cancer-specific survival

The relapse and specific survival analyses were carried out within a mean follow-up time of 17.7 months. The shortest and longest follow-up times were three and 46 months, respectively, and corresponded to patients in the pT2-3 group.

Only miR-21 was significantly associated with relapse-free survival in low-grade pTa tumors. Patients with miRNA expression levels less than or equal to 1.08 survived disease-free for an average of 24.6 months. In contrast, those with expression above 1.08 remained disease-free for only 16.3 months, demonstrating that higher expression of miR-21 was related to higher recurrence rates (p = 0.02) (Figure 8).

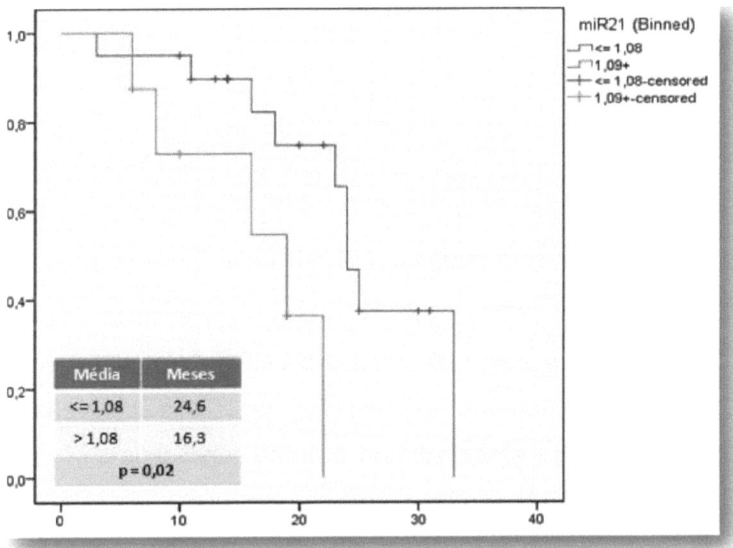

Figura 8 - Kaplan-Meyer curve showing the difference in SLR of low-grade pTa tumors in relation to miR-21 expression

miR-10a was associated with both recurrence-free survival and cancer-specific survival in high-grade invasive tumors. Patients with expression levels greater than 0.23 showed shorter RLS and DFS, with a mean time of 13 and 15.3 months, respectively. On the other hand, expression profiles lower than or equal to 0.23 were associated with better RLS and DFS, with mean survival times of 26.1 and 27.3 months respectively. These behavioral patterns led to statistical differences for RLS (p= 0.007) and SCE (p = 0.04) in relation to miR-10a (Figure 9).

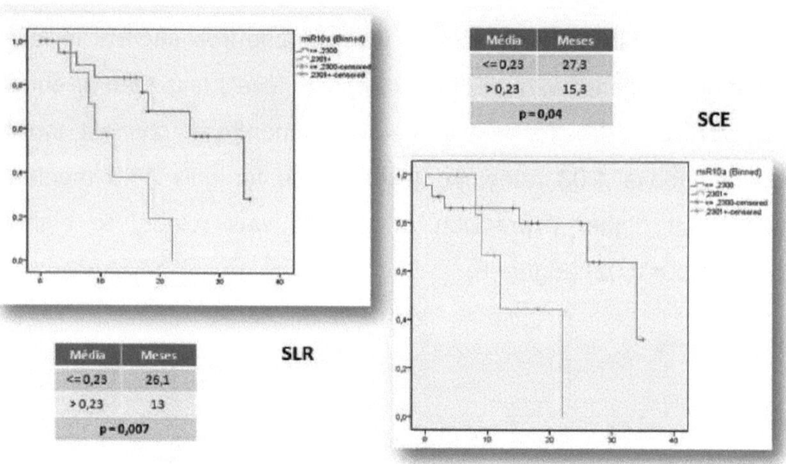

Figura 9 - Kaplan-Meyer curve showing the differences in SLR and SCE for miR-10a in high-grade pT2-3 tumors

Considering miR-145, levels above 0.66 correlated with shorter relapse-free survival for pT2-3 tumors (average of 15.6 months), while expressions less than or equal to 0.66 were associated with an average survival time of 25.2 months (p = 0.03) (Figure 10).

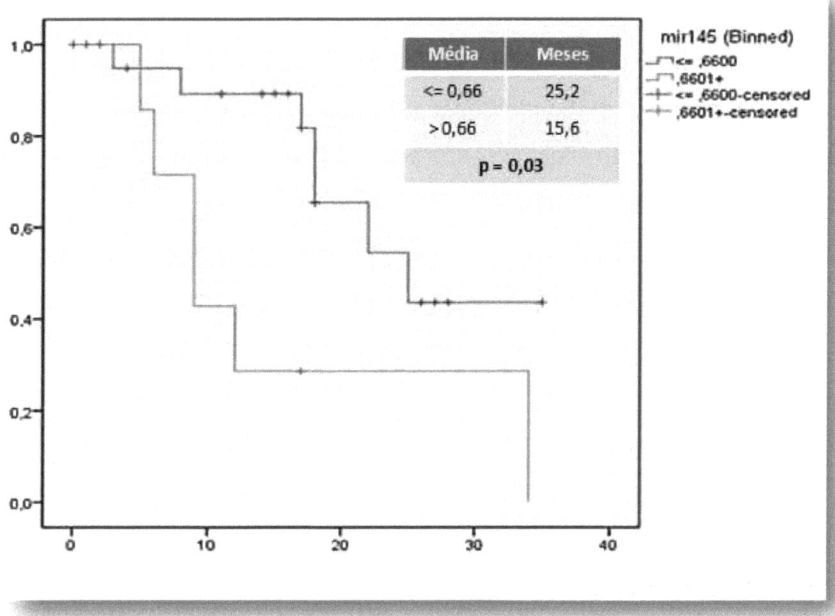

Figura 10 - Kaplan-Meyer curve showing differences in SLR in high-grade pT2-3 tumors in relation to miR-145 expression

5. Discussion

Currently, more than 1,400 miRNAs have been identified which, regulating approximately one third of human genes (Lewis et al., 2005), appear to play a fundamental role in the physiological and pathological processes of organs and tissues (Bartel and Chen, 2004).

The findings here are in line with the literature. With the exception of miR-10a for low-grade pTa and miR-100, 21 and 205 in high-grade pT2-3 tumors, which were overexpressed in more than half of the cases, all the others were underexpressed in both tumor groups. This is relevant and demonstrates that human miRNAs act mainly as tumor suppressors (Gottardo et al., 2007; Neely et al., 2008; Leite et al., 2009; Ichimi et al., 2009; Veerla et al., 2009; Catto et al., 2009; Sachdeva et al., 2009; Chiyomaru et al., 2010; Dip et al., 2011).

Our main objective was to identify miRNA expression signatures that could corroborate the characterization of the two specific groups of urothelial carcinoma, both from a molecular and behavioral point of view. When we considered two tumor groups defined by different grade and stage, we identified expression differences in only four miRNA (miR-100, miR-10a, miR-21 and miR-205) of the 14 studied, with different expression behaviors in both groups. These profiles seem to define each tumor group and can separate them in a very specific way.

miR-100 was under-expressed in all low-grade carcinomas, pTa and has been shown to be under-expressed in ovarian carcinoma and squamous cell carcinoma of the oral cavity (Nagaraja et al., 2010; Henson et al., 2009). In urothelial carcinoma, miR-100 may have as its main target the FGFR3 gene, whose mutation and increased activity is related to this neoplasm. Under physiological conditions, miR-100 negatively regulates FGFR3, thus decreasing its expression levels in a post transcriptional manner. Our data show that there may be an alternative pathway for the carcinogenesis of low-grade urothelial carcinomas other than the FGFR3 activating mutation. The under-expression of miR-100 that we found in 100% of the tumors could be responsible for the over-expression of FGFR3 and the development of low-grade carcinoma. Catto et al. (2009) found an inversely proportional relationship between miR-100 and FGFR3, where the under-expression of miRNA led to increased gene activity before the mutation occurred, suggesting that the increased concentration of FGFR3 would facilitate the mutational event through increased cell *turnover* or the natural selection of mutant cells. Perhaps the loss of miR-100 expression is the first triggering event of the disease and could occur long before its clinical appearance. The importance of this fact is that it allows for the predictability of conservative treatment, bladder preservation due to the rare chances of progression and excellent survival. We can suggest that miR-100 expression measurements could be used in clinical practice as a possible diagnostic and prognostic marker for low-grade CUB pTa.

On the other hand, most invasive tumors were associated with overexpression of miR-100 (56,7%). It is speculated that it acts as

negative controller of the THAP-2 gene, directly involved in the control of cell proliferation through the modulation of proteins that control the cell cycle such as pRB and E2F (Bessière et al., 2008). The loss of function of the RB1, p53 and PTEN genes is involved in the carcinogenic pathway of invasive tumors, promoting genomic instability and facilitating their progression (Figure 1). The overexpression of miR-100 in pT2-3 could promote the silencing of THAP-2 and, consequently, RB1. The BAZ2A and SMARCA5 genes are also targets of miR-100 and are associated with DNA transcriptional repression and chromosomal instability (Zhou *et al.*, 2002; Bozhenok *et al.*, 2002). However, these genes have not yet been studied in CUB and require further research to prove their role in bladder carcinogenesis.

For miR-10a, we found overexpression in 73.3% of pTa tumors compared to only 6.7% of pT2-3 tumors. miR-10a is located on chromosome 17q21, within the HOXB gene *cluster*, between the HOXB-4 and HOXB-5 genes, and probably plays a regulatory role in cell differentiation (Garzon et al., 2006; Huang et al., 2010; Foley et al., 2011). In addition to the usual pattern of action on the 3' untranslated region of the mRNA, miR-10a can bind to the 5' region of the mRNA and increase the translation of ribosomal proteins, positively regulating global protein translation (Orom et al., 2008). These interactions could exert a proliferative stimulus, affecting the ability to differentiate and promoting cell transformation, characteristic of neoplasms in general.

Our results are consistent with those published by Veerla et al. (2009). In that study, the authors showed that miR-10a expression was 2.47 times higher in non-invasive pTa tumors than in invasive pT1 and pT2-3 tumors. Even without establishing a mechanistic relationship between miR-10a and the FGFR3 gene, the authors speculate an association between them, which could be fundamental to the carcinogenesis of CUB, pTa.

Although some current studies show an oncogenic role for the miR-10 family in other human neoplasms, miR-10a can have a very broad function, depending on the type of tumor and its genetic-molecular characteristics. For example, Ma et al. (2007) and Weiss et al. (2009) observed an oncogenic role for miR-10 in breast and pancreatic cancer, with its overexpression being directly associated with greater tumor aggressiveness, the development of metastases and a worse prognosis. Agirre et al. (2008) showed a relationship between the under-expression of this miRNA and increased cell proliferation and progression of chronic myeloid leukemia.

Although overexpression of miR-10a is related to low-grade, non-invasive tumors, we showed that lower expression of miR-10a was associated with almost double the recurrence-free survival and cancer-specific survival. Garzon et al. (2006) described the under-expression of miR-10a in relation to the over-expression of the HOXA-1 gene and consequent cell differentiation. We could therefore suggest that the greater the under-expression of miRNA, the greater the expression of HOXA-1 and the differentiation of the neoplastic cell, leading to better tumor behavior.

miR-21 was markedly overexpressed in invasive high-grade tumors, being almost 17 times higher than in non-invasive tumors (pTa = 1.08 vs pT2/pT3 = 18.17; p = 0.02). The same was described by Neely et al. (2008) who showed a 10-fold increase in miR-21 expression in high-grade invasive CUB. Current evidence establishes miR-21 as a truly oncogenic miRNA, overexpressed in the vast majority of tumors. It is capable of promoting tumorigenesis by increasing cell proliferation and blocking apoptotic control mechanisms. The same was found by Si et al. (2006) in breast cancer.

miR-21 indirectly targets the p53 gene, considered to be the most important gene involved in the carcinogenesis of invasive CUB (Esrig et al., 1994). p53 is a gene responsible for controlling the cell's global activities through cell cycle inhibition, apoptosis induction and DNA repair. Catto *et al.* (2009) observed overexpression of miR-21 associated with inactivation of the p53 gene, linking it to tumor invasion and progression.

PTEN is another important gene involved in the carcinogenic pathways of CUB and is also a target of miR-21 (Wu, 2009; McConkey et al., 2010; Meng et al., 2007). PTEN is a lipid phosphatase that suppresses the PI3K/AKT carcinogenic pathway and blocks cell growth, characterizing it as a classic tumor suppressor gene. In a current review of the genetic-molecular mechanisms involved in the initiation and progression of CUB, McConkey et al. (2010) suggest that loss of PTEN function is much more common in invasive CUB related to inactivation of the PTEN/PI3K/AKT/mTOR pathway, characterizing a worse prognostic factor.

We also showed that overexpression of miR-21 was associated with worse relapse-free survival in pTa tumors, and that the OSL was 51% higher for cases with expression levels less than or equal to 1.08 (16.3 versus 24.6 months). This fact strengthens the oncogenic characteristics of miR-21 presented in this study.

All the other miRNAs were underexpressed in both groups of tumors.

All pTa tumors and 63.3% of pT2-3 tumors showed under-expression of miR-205. Although almost two-thirds of the high-grade invasive tumors showed under-expression of miRNA, the average expression levels of the 30 cases tended towards relatively considerable over-expression (6.91). miR-205 has been defined as a tumor suppressor and is involved in epithelial-mesenchymal transition (EMT), the process by which a malignant neoplasm is able to carry out a fundamental step in tumor progression, i.e. dissemination to other organs. miR-205, like the miR-200 family, physiologically inhibits classic E-cadherin suppressor genes (ZEB-1 and ZEB-2), an adhesion molecule responsible for maintaining the epithelium with its usual physiological characteristics (Gregory et al., 2008). The loss of expression of miR-205 allows the hyperactivity of ZEB-1 and ZEB-2 which, in turn, suppress the functions of E-cadherin, thus allowing the epithelial disjunction that facilitates the metastasis process. EMT is crucial for the maintenance and success of the neoplastic process and is directly related to worse behavior, greater tumor aggressiveness and, consequently, worse prognosis and shorter survival. The role of miR-205 is practically the same in various types of human tumors, which is to hinder their dissemination. Some authors have demonstrated its under-expression in non-small cell lung cancer, breast cancer and prostate cancer (Lebanony et al., 2009; Wu et al., 2009; Gandellini et al., 2009).

In CUB, aberrant hypermethylation of promoter regions on chromosome 1q32.2, the location of the gene that produces miR-205, has been shown (Wiklund et al., 2011). In 2008, Neely et al. established that the miR-21/miR-205 ratio progressively increases with tumor progression. Very interestingly, Brabletz and Brabletz (2010) demonstrated that the ZEB/miR-200 autoregulatory loop is crucial for defining the state of the cell. Thus, when the loop is in favor of ZEB, the progressive state prevails and tumor spread occurs beyond the epithelial barriers. On the other hand, when it is in favor of the miR-200 family, the proliferative state prevails, leading to tumor growth. According to the authors, neoplastic tissue needs both states, i.e. an initial proliferative state that will make the tumour grow, and a later progressive state, responsible for the metastasization process. Interestingly, the under-expression of miR-200 would favor the process of dissemination, but once the metastasis sites have been defined, proliferation will have to take place again, which is why the re-expression of miR-200 is necessary.

These conditions are exactly those demonstrated here for miR-205, a miRNA similar to the miR-200 family. What we observed was its under-expression in 100% of pTa tumors, consistent with the initial proliferative carcinogenic state. At the same time, one third of the pT2-3 tumors were overexpressed and the levels of under-expression in the remaining cases were lower than in the pTa tumors. These findings suggest a progressive phenotype and the re-expression of miR-205 is probably tending towards a return to the proliferative state that occurs after dissemination.

We observed a global loss of miR-let7c expression in both pTa (86.7%) and pT2/pT3 (93.3%) tumors. This fact highlights the suppressive role of this miRNA, consolidated in practically all the neoplasms where it has been studied, and reflects its fundamental action in protecting against malignant events. The RAS and c-MYC oncogenes are targets of miR-let7c and their under-expression is related to neoplastic development (Reinhart et al., 2000; Johnson et al., 2005). RAS is the second most important oncogene in the tumorigenesis of low-grade pTa (Wu, 2005). Single mutations lead to gene alterations which, in turn, promote an exaggerated stimulation of the AKT and STAT pathways, generating a high rate of cell proliferation. c- MYC is the prototype oncogene, its role is to inhibit RB1 (Reinhart et al., 2000) and is associated with the CUB pT2-3. c-MYC is capable of stimulating the cyclins CDK4, CDK6 and D1, promoting the phosphorylation and inactivation of RB1 with consequent mitogenic and proliferative stimulation. On the other hand, c-MYC can increase the function of p53 via inhibition of MDM-2, favoring cell cycle arrest and apoptosis (Knowles, 2008).

Similarly, miR-125b was under-expressed in 100% of pTa cases and 93.3% of pT2-3 cases. The role of miR-125b is controversial in the literature. Studies define it as a tumor suppressor miRNA and therefore under-expressed, while others classify it as an oncogenic miRNA (Ichimi et al., 2009; Le et al., 2009; Klussmann et al., 2010; Rajabi et al., 2010; Liang et al., 2010). Studying ovarian tumors, Guan et al. (2011) observed a protective role for miR-125b where it was found to be under-expressed, and its reintroduction prevented tumor formation in *nude* mice infected with human ovarian neoplastic cells. On the other hand, Shi et al. (2011) demonstrated the oncogenic role of miR-125b in prostate cancer, since it targets pro-apoptotic genes (p53, Puma and Bak-1).

In agreement with our findings, Huang et al. (2011) demonstrated under-expression of miR-125b in bladder tumors and in CUB cell lines. miR-125b could suppress bladder tumorigenesis by silencing the transcription factor E2F3, which is fundamental to the cell cycle. The authors found an inverse relationship between them, and the transfection of miR-125b into cell cultures was able to reverse the proliferative effects by reducing E2F3 levels. Another target of miR-125b is the KRT-7 gene, which is involved in the process of DNA replication, cytoskeleton organization and regulation of translation, and is an overexpressed oncogene (Ichimi et al., 2009).

pTa and pT2-3 tumors showed under-expression of miR-143 (96.7% for both groups) and miR-145 (73.3% and 86.7%, respectively),

suggesting tumor suppressor functions and control of the cell's normal activities. These miRNAs are located very close together on chromosome 5q32 and share the same tumor suppressor function. There is evidence of the action of miR-143 on RAS. As already discussed, mutated RAS leads to stimulation of the MAPK/AKT/STAT pathways, which triggers the development of low-grade pTa (Wu, 2009) and may also be involved in the pathways of high-grade tumors (McConkey et al., 2010). Lin et al. (2009) demonstrated by studying neoplastic tissues and CUB cell lines that under-expression of miR-143 is the rule in these neoplasms. In tumor tissues, miR-143 was 13.7 times lower than in the normal control. In the EJ and T24 tumor cell lines, miR-143 was not identified and when transfected into the cultures, it significantly inhibited cell growth.

With regard to miR-145, several studies have validated this miRNA as an inhibitor of the cell cycle and cell growth and an inducer of apoptosis, reducing the possibility of invasion and the development of metastases. miR-145 is under-expressed in colon, lung, breast and prostate cancer, among others (Ozen et al., 2008; Izzoti et al., 2009; Sachdeva et al., 2009). Our results are consistent with the findings in the literature and show a marked under-expression of miRNA in both tumor groups.

Sachdeva and Mo (2010) showed in breast cancer lines that the mucin 1 gene (MUC-1) gene was involved in initiation, invasion and

miR-145 is able to inhibit these characteristics, controlling neoplastic development. Another target of miR-145 is the c-MYC gene (Sachdeva et al., 2009), an oncogene involved in the carcinogenic process of invasive CUB (Knowles, 2008). The p53 gene is an inducer of miR-145 and is directly related to the carcinogenesis of high-grade invasive BUC. In 2009, Sachdeva et al. observed that, under physiological conditions, higher levels of p53 due to cellular stress led to an increase in miR-145 concentrations through the p53 response element (p53RE). miR-145, in turn, blocks the activity of c-MYC (a negative regulator of p21), and the loss of miRNA expression may promote failure in the regulation of this oncogene, decrease p21 levels and increase cell proliferation. In addition, the PI3K/AKT carcinogenic pathway is capable of stimulating the production of miR-145. Interruption of these complex mechanisms mediated by the under-expression of miR-145 could lead to, or at least initiate, CUB carcinogenesis (Sachdeva and Mo, 2010). Following the same idea, Spizzo et al. (2010) analyzing breast cancer cell lines, demonstrated the crucial suppressive role of miR-145, and its transfection prevented cell growth and proliferation and induced p53-mediated apoptosis. p53 can also trigger the miRNA enzymatic machinery, mainly RNAse III Drosha, and thus stimulate the production of several miRNAs, including miR-145. Loss of p53 function due to mutations would generate inadequate production of miR-145 and its consequent under-expression (Suzuki et al., 2009). Chiyomaru et al. (2010) demonstrated in CUB an association between the FSCN-1 oncogene and the silencing promoted by miR-

145 and suggest that the loss of miRNA expression generally related to bladder tumors of all stages allows for the loss of FSCN-1 silencing and greater aggressiveness and tumor invasion capacity.

We found an association between miR-145 and recurrence-free survival for high-grade invasive tumors. Patients survived disease-free for a mean time of 15.6 months when expression values were above 0.66, while this time was 61.5% longer for values less than or equal to the cut-off point (25.2 months). Despite the statistical difference found ($p = 0.03$), higher expression levels were associated with more recurrence and this is not in line with the rationale proposed for miRNA, a true tumor suppressor. We expected that higher concentrations of miR-145 would correlate with better tumor behavior and prognosis, and what we can speculate here is that perhaps, faced with the major disorganization of the cellular machinery due to the loss of function of p53, the cell increases the production of miR-145 by mechanisms other than that mediated by p53. This could be seen as a reactionary cellular event in an attempt to maintain the physiological conditions of the neoplastic cell.

Eighty percent of pTa tumors and 90% of pT2-3 tumors showed under-expression of miR-221, and there seems to be a trend towards greater under-expression as tumor grade and staging increase. While the literature demonstrates an oncogenic role for miR-221 (Sage et al., 2007; Lu et al., 2010), here we demonstrate discordant results and hypothesize that miR- 221 has a tumor suppressor function in CUB. Pineau et al. (2010) demonstrated overexpression of miR-221 in hepatocarcinoma (HCC) and suggested its action on p27KIP1 (cyclin inhibitor and cell cycle suppressor) and DDIT4 (negative regulator of mTOR).

miR-223 was under-expressed in pTa and pT2-3 tumors (96.7% and 66.7%, respectively). The levels of under-expression were more evident in non-invasive pTa tumors, but there were no differences between the groups. This miRNA is under-expressed in chronic lymphocytic leukemias (CLL), with the higher the levels of under-expression, the greater the tumor volume, the aggressiveness of the disease and the presence of worse prognostic factors (Stamatopoulos et al., 2009). Wong et al. (2008) showed that miR-223 is under-expressed in HCC and that its restoration in cell culture inhibits cell viability by silencing the oncoprotein Statmina-1 (STMN-1). In ovarian tumors, miR-223 is overexpressed in recurrent neoplasms compared to primary neoplasms (Laios et al., 2008). Chen et al. (2008), analyzing miRNA in plasma, found overexpression of miR-223 in patients with non-small cell lung cancer.

In contrast to our findings, Gottardo et al. (2007), studying CUB of different grades and stages, found that miR-223 expression was on average 1.5 times higher in the tumor than in normal tissue.

Half of the patients with pTa tumors showed under-expression of miR-15a, while 53.3% of the pT2-3 tumors did. Under-expression of miR- 16-1 occurred in the majority of pTa and pT2-3 tumors (73.3% for both groups), with no differences for either miRNA when comparing the two groups for histological grade ($p = 0.78$ and $p = 0.81$) and staging ($p = 0.93$ and $p = 0.95$). miR-15a and 16-1 showed the most heterogeneous results of all the miRNAs studied. There seems to be no pattern of behavior for them in CUB, which could suggest that these miRNAs are not involved in bladder carcinogenesis. These two suppressor miRNAs are related to the development of chronic lymphocytic leukemia by acting on the BCL-2 oncogene (Calin et al., 2002; Cimmino et al., 2005), which does not seem to play a role in bladder carcinogenesis.

miR-199a was also under-expressed in both tumor groups (93.3% for pTa and 83.3% for pT2-3), with no significant differences observed for prognostic factors. The same was described by Ichimi et

al. (2008) in CUB. Low levels of miR-199a have already been described in ovarian, testicular, HCC and osteosarcoma tumors (Chen et al., 2008; Cheung et al., 2011; Fornari et al., 2010; Duan et al., 2011) and miRNA seems to be directly involved in tumor progression, being related to a worse prognosis of these neoplasms. Fornari et al. (2010) studying HCC suggested mTOR as a target of miR-199a, demonstrating an inverse relationship between them. As with HCC, the PI3K/AKT/mTOR pathway is also involved in the carcinogenesis of high-grade invasive CUB and the under-expression of miR-199a could explain the over-stimulation of mTOR production and, at least in part, tumor establishment and progression. Cheung et al. (2011) found that the PODXL gene, which produces an anti-adhesive protein present in aggressive tumors, is overexpressed in testicular cancer and is the target of miR-199a, which is under-expressed due to hypermethylation of its producer region. Both Chen and Cheung carried out transfection studies of miR-199a in tumor cell cultures and observed inhibition of cell growth, suggesting its use in the treatment of these neoplasms.

The marked under-expression of miR-452 in both tumor groups (93.3% in the pTa group and 96.7% in the pT2-3 group) allows us to assume that this miRNA plays a tumor suppressor role in CUB. Furthermore, the increasing levels of underexpression and the higher percentage of underexpressed cases as histological grade and tumor stage evolve reinforce this role, since the greater the aggressiveness, the lower the levels of miR-452 expression. Our findings contradict those published for CUB. Veerla et al. (2009) studied 14 patients, 50% of whom had positive lymph nodes, and showed that overexpression of miR-452 was related to the presence of lymph node metastases. On the other hand, Mascaux et al. (2009), evaluating bronchial squamous cell carcinoma, found a loss of miR-452 expression related to poor tumor behavior. Human miR-452 has approximately 220 target genes and, among them, two that are directly involved in cell growth and proliferation (E2F3 and MEF2C) and which could no longer be inhibited by miR-452 in CUB. This assumption merits further mechanistic studies.

Although some factors such as the small number of cases and the short follow-up time may have been limiting, our study was able to demonstrate a difference in the expression of four miRNAs in low-grade, pTa and high-grade, pT2-3 tumors that can be incorporated into the molecular pathways already described. We suggest that this expression profile could be used as a prognostic indicator and help urologists and oncologists choose the best therapeutic approach.

This characterization can also be used to develop target drugs, such as the instillation of miR-100 in BCG-resistant low-grade pTa carcinomas.

More extensive studies and experimental proof of the action of the different miRNAs described in this study are needed to better understand the role of these molecules in urothelial bladder carcinoma.

5.1 Final considerations

This preliminary study has allowed us to reflect on the true functions of the miRNAs studied here, not only because of their wide-ranging action capacities, but also because of their ability to define the fate of the cell. Considering the promising findings here and in the face of a "world" not yet discovered about these fantastic molecules, we intend to study the carcinogenic pathways involved in CUB in detail, in an attempt to identify their key events, introducing miRNAs as their fundamental components. This will allow us to speculate on their roles as potential diagnostic and prognostic markers and to develop miRNA targets for molecular therapeutic intervention. In addition, we want to measure miRNA in urine and, if possible, make it a non-invasive test and easy to acquire the material to be studied, regardless of the need for tumor samples.

Through this new line of research set up by our laboratory, we will have the opportunity to develop more complete analyses of the pathways of invasive and non-invasive tumors by means of mechanistic studies of transfection/inhibition in cell culture, immunohistochemical analysis, the luciferase method, Western Blotting and DNA sequencing of the genes involved, which will allow a broader understanding of these processes and, certainly, better management of this very prevalent disease.

Finally, the future of anti-tumor molecular target therapy will probably be based not on one, but on a group of miRNAs that will work together in the various stages of the tumor process and will be able to identify the disease, predict its behavior and control it or definitely treat it effectively.

6. Conclusion

Most of the miRNAs were underexpressed in low-grade and high-grade bladder urothelial carcinoma, pTa and pT2-3.

Comparing low-grade pTa carcinomas and high-grade pT2-3 carcinomas, we found a difference in the expression levels of miR-100, miR-10a, miR-21 and miR-205.

Low-grade carcinomas, pTa, showed under-expression of miR- 100, miR-21 and miR-205, while miR-10a was over-expressed. In high-grade carcinoma, pT2-3, the pattern was exactly the opposite, i.e. there was overexpression of miR-100, miR-21 and miR-205 and underexpression of miR-10a. These profiles distinguish the two tumor groups and could be used as diagnostic and prognostic biomarkers.

miR-10a and miR-145 were able to secrete relapse-free survival in pT2-3 tumors and their higher expressions translated into higher relapse rates. The same is true for miR-21 in pTa tumors.

miR-10a was associated with cancer-specific survival in pT2-3 tumors and higher levels of miRNA reflected higher mortality from bladder urothelial carcinoma.

7. ANNEXES

Annex A - Informed Consent Form

HOSPITAL DAS CLiNICAS DA FACULDADE DE MEDICINA DA UNIVERSITY OF SÀO PAULO-HCFMUSP

1. IDENTIFICATION DATA OF THE RESEARCH SUBJECT OR LEGAL RESPONSIBILITY

A.NAME: ____

IDENTITY DOCUMENT NO. : SEX : M □ F □

DATE OF BIRTH:

ADDRESS: ____

BAIRRO: ________________________

CITY:__________________________

PHONE: ________________________

B. LEGAL GUARDIAN:__________________________________

NATURE (degree of kinship, guardian, curator, etc.):_______________

ID CARD : .... SEX: M □ F □

DATE OF BIRTH: _____________

ADDRESS: ____

BAIRRO: ___________________

CITY:_____________________

PHONE: ___________________

2. RESEARCH DATA

A. TITLE OF RESEARCH PROTOCOL: Characterization of MicroRNA Expression in Invasive Urothelial Carcinoma of the Bladder

B. RESEARCHER : Drª. Kàtia Ramos Moreira Leite

C. POSITION: Doctor, head of the Medical Research Laboratory of the Urology Discipline - LIM/55

D. REGISTRATION REGIONAL COUNCIL: N° 51442

E. HCFMUSP UNIT: Department of Surgery, Discipline of Urology

F. RESEARCH RISK ASSESSMENT:

MiNIMOX RISK MEDIUM RISK □

LOW RISK □ HIGHER RISK □

G. DURATION OF RESEARCH: 24 months

3. GUIDELINES

1 - The aim of this study is to evaluate a new marker for diagnosing and/or defining the prognosis of bladder cancer.

2 - The work will be carried out using part of the tissue that was removed during your surgery, and will not cause any harm to you or to the material itself, which will remain preserved for your future interest.

3 - No additional procedures will be necessary.

4-Therefore, this research does not bring you any discomfort or risk. 5 - There is no direct benefit for you, only at the end of the study will we be able to conclude the presence of any benefit for the patients, which could be a new tool for discovering or ruling out the hypothesis of bladder cancer, or even defining the degree of malignancy of your tumor.

6 - As there are no additional procedures to be carried out, there are no alternative procedures.

7 - Guaranteed access: at any stage of the study, you will have access to the professionals responsible for the research to clarify any doubts you may have. The principal investigator is Dr. ***Kâtia Ramos Moreira Leite***, who can be reached at Av. Dr. Enéas de Carvalho Aguiar 255- 7° andar sala 710-F,

Telephone (011) 3069 - 8080. If you have any considerations or doubts about the ethics of the research, please contact the Research Ethics Committee (CEP) - Rua Ovidio Pires de Campos, 225 - 5° andar - tel: 3069-6442 ext. 16, 17, 18 or 20, FAX: 3069-6442 ext. 26 - E-mail: cappesq@hcnet.usp.br

8 - You are guaranteed the freedom to withdraw your consent at any time and to stop participating in the study, without any prejudice to the continuity of your treatment. at the Institution;

9 9 - Right to confidentiality - The information obtained will be analyzed together with other patients, and the identification of any patient will not be disclosed. patient;

10 - The right to be kept up to date on the partial results of research, when in open studies, or results that are known to of researchers;

11 - Expenses and compensation: there are no personal expenses for the participant at any stage of the study, including examinations and consultations. There is also no financial compensation related to your participation. If there are any additional expenses, they will be absorbed by the research budget.

12 - The researcher's commitment to use the data and material collected only for this research.

I believe that I have been sufficiently informed about the information that I have read or that has been read to me describing the study: "Characterization of MicroRNA Expression in Invasive Urothelial Carcinoma of the Bladder". I discussed my decision to participate in this study with Dr ***Kàtia Ramos Moreira Leite***. It was made clear to me what the purposes of the study are, the procedures to be carried out, their discomforts and risks, the guarantees of confidentiality and ongoing clarification. It is also clear that my participation is free of charge and that I have guaranteed access to hospital treatment when necessary. I voluntarily agree to take part in this study and may withdraw my consent at any time, before or during the study, without penalty or loss of any benefit I may have acquired, or in my care at this service.

Signature of patient/legal representative

Date / /

Signature of witness

Date / /

For patients under the age of 18, who are illiterate, semi-literate or have a hearing or visual impairment.

I declare that I have properly and voluntarily obtained the Free and Informed Consent of this patient or legal representative to participate in this study.

Dr. Kâtia Ramos Moreira Leite Date / /

(responsible for the study)

Annex B - Protocol for Extracting miRNA from Frozen Tissue - mirVana™ miRNA Isolation Kit (Ambion®)

1. Measure or estimate the weight of the sample
2. Macerate the tissue in liquid nitrogen or macerator
3. Add 10 volumes of lysis solution (Lysis/Binding Buffer)
4. Add 1/10 of the volume of the homogenate additive
5. Leave the mixture on ice for 10 minutes
6. Add a volume of Acid- phenol:chloroform equal to the volume of the lysis solution.
7. Vortex 30-60 seconds
8. Centrifuge for 5 minutes at 10,000 rpm at room temperature
9. Carefully remove the aqueous phase and transfer to a new tube; note the

volume removed

10. Add 1/3 of the volume of 100% ethanol

11. Vortex or invert the tube

12. Transfer the sample to the column (maximum volume 700 μL)

13. Centrifuge for 15 seconds at 10,000 rpm at room temperature

14. Collect the FILTRATE and transfer to a new tube; note the total volume; the filter contains RNA and the filtrate the small RNA

15. Add 2/3 of the volume of 100% ethanol to the filtrate and mix.

16. Transfer the filtrate to a new filter (maximum volume 700 μL)

17. Centrifuge for 15 seconds at 10,000 rpm at room temperature

18. Discard the filtrate (the miRNAs are now in the filter)

19. Add 700 μL of wash solution 1 and centrifuge for 5-10 seconds

20. Add 700 μL of wash solution 2/3 and centrifuge for 5-10 seconds (1ª time)

21. Add 700 μL of wash solution 2/3 and centrifuge for 5-10 seconds (2nd time).

22. After discarding the filtrate, centrifuge the empty tubes for 1 minute at 10,000 rpm at room temperature to dry and remove residues.

23. Transfer the filter to a new tube and add 100 μL of $H2O$ pre-heated to 95° C (Elution Solution) and close the tube.

24. Centrifuge 10,000 rpm at room temperature for 20-30 seconds

25. Quantify the samples and store in a freezer - 20 °C

Annex C - Expression values of the 14 miRNAs studied for each low-grade pTa tumor sample

miRNA pTa	100	21	Let7c	125b	143	145	221	223	15a	16-1	199a	10a	452	205
B54	0,117	0,211	0,103	0.505	0,018	0.422	0,003	0,002	0,16	$2,6^{ns}$	0,29	761,2	39,87	0,35
B56	0,440	0,167	0,003	0,4	0,018	0,090	0,61	0,135	0,21	0,04	0,03	113,8	0,0001	0,005
B61	0,198	0,029	0,013	0,085	0,002	0,144	4,61	0,554	13,57	2,33	0,05	197,4	0,002	0,005
B74	0,072	0,040	0,05	0 128	0,002	0,023	0,392	0,132	1,32	0,001	0,01	16,11	0,007	0,036
B75	0,083	0,022	0,034	0 123	0,002	0,033	0,307	0,285	0,32	1,89	0,04	3,194	0,0003	0,077
B79	0,0009	0,029	0,206	0 113	0,008	0,288	0,14	0,103	0,32	1,11	0,26	2,271	0,008	0,058

B87	8,9-'3	0,414	13,14	0,334	4,13	2,275	2,01	0,711	2,18	6,04	2,7	6,282	0,04	0,005
B91	1,2"12	2,890	12,85	0.262	0,31	9,037	1,942	0,758	4,65	12,3	0,78	37,74	0,08	0,006
B95	3,1-"	0,566	2,29	0 152	0,351	24,06	0,296	0,06	0,77	0,95	0,66	9,159	0,04	0,019
B102	0,0007	0,373	1,234	0,12	0,228	3,947	0,452	0,098	0,48	0,56	0,63	7,156	0,02	0,025
B107	0,0008	0,393	0,115	0,017	0,036	0,552	0,489	0,136	0,28	0,66	0,18	32,22	0,02	0,034
BW	0,007	1,433	0,434	0 133	0,063	1,428	1,18	0,074	0,53	1,24	0,78	6,005	0,05	0,03
B112	0,0007	0,710	0,0003	0,053	0,036	0,711	17,64	9,494	6,58	0,95	0,06	114,3	0,06	0,002
B118	0,0003	0,018	6,3"4	9,4"s	0,01	0,324	0,503	0,003	1,62	0,06	0,01	0,149	0,04	0,102
B121	0,001	0,026	0,003	0 147	0,11	1,021	0,151	0,033	2,42	0,24	0,09	0,916	0,007	0,189
B147	0,0008	1,264	0,005	0,042	0,012	0,035	0,627	0,073	4,55	0,61	0,05	12,92	0,001	0,043
B161	0,008	5,849	0,029	0,086	0,082	0,407	0,301	0,139	11,09	2,21	0,19	7,745	0,12	0,058
B163	2,8-'	1,158	0,021	0,062	0,009	0,148	0,351	0,174	4,23	0,91	0,2	3,746	0,02	0,043
B164	6,1"1o	0,882	0,016	0,02	0,0008	0,026	0,212	0,018	0,46	0,52	0,08	2,302	0,02	0,101
B169	3,4^8	0,926	0,013	0,081	0,003	0,248	0,133	0,054	1,73	0,58	0,16	2,447	0,08	0,099
B170	2,8"8	0,655	0,025	0,051	0,001	0,065	0,12	0,01	0,5	0,5	0,09	1,406	0,06	0,105
B193	1,2"7	1,666	0,162	0 154	0,002	0,126	0,278	0,011	0,74	0,8	0,19	0,543	0,6	0,055
4	2,1"8	1,144	0,008	0,032	0,0007	0,044	0,075	0,002	0,51	0,51	0,06	2,425	0,09	0,078
24	1,3"β	11,13	0,182	0.762	0,023	1,701	0,994	0,189	15,3	8,64	1,5	30,80	1,04	0,004
25	2"8	0,002	0,041	0,018	0,002	1,000	2,573	0,951	2,75	0,18	0,03	18,49	0,01	0,002
31	0,073	0,540	0,02	0,661	0,006	0,001	0,009	0,466	1,64	0,21	1,06	0,031	0,007	0,011
MB2	0,023	0,005	0,009	0,014	0,016	0,120	0,01	0,146	0,7	0,006	0,0008	0,004	0,23	0,24
MB6	0,109	0,002	0,008	0,0004	0,0004	0,039	0,147	0,012	2,92	0,009	0,001	0,193	0,005	0,032
MB9	0,001	0,005	0,0009	0,0002	0,0002	0,017	0,007	0,005	0,18	0,003	0,001	0,078	0,002	0,152
MB12	0,003	0,004	0,003	0,003	7,4"5	0,023	0,025	0,003	0,1	0,005	0,5	0,157	0,005	0,024

Annex D - Expression values of the 14 miRNAs studied for each high-grade pT2-3 tumor sample

miRNA pT2-3	100	21	Let7c	125b	143	145	221	223	15a	16-1	199a	10a	452	205
B53	0,505	1,780	0,108	0,09	0,07	0,129	0,348	0,27	0,29	0,6	0,02	0,001	0,005	1,954
B59	18,93	56,50	0,001	0,012	0,35	10,25	0,543	3,888	0,6	3,3	0,67	0,922	0,001	0,604
B60	0,024	6,432	0,0003	0,002	0,006	0,906	0,107	0,054	3,74	0.72	0,3	0,228	0,001	1,931
B 64	1,593	10,33	0.04	0,0006	0,074	0,675	0,073	1,94	4,28	0.97	0,69	0,407	0,01	0,241
B70	9,136	12,45	1,322	0,266	0,096	2,080	0,335	2,236	4,51	1.45	6,78	1,266	0,01	0,697
B71	1,29	1,928	0,125	0,036	0,028	0,126	0,134	0,491	0,69	0.24	1,46	0,071	0,005	1,083
B81	0,151	0,233	0,009	0,013	0,0003	0,215	0,171	6,203	0,69	0,6	0,03	0,085	0,004	0,926
B93	0,074	1,090	0.59	0,176	0,015	0,187	0,393	3,09	1,74	0,001	0,87	0,052	0,07	0,06
1	1,954	0,611	0.644	0,197	0,107	0,153	0,087	0,913	0,25	0.38	2,9	0,044	0,006	0,515
5	0,395	0,600	0,024	0,073	0,036	0,065	0,209	1,97	0,64	0,4	0,73	0,004	0,08	1,41
B97	21,08	0,593	0,614	0,31	3.85	0,034	0,514	1,541	1,88	2,37	0,03	0,242	0,02	0,351
B99	22,48	0,153	0,011	0,054	0,163	0,008	0,064	0,78	0,5	0,63	0,04	0,01	0,14	6,491
B117	520,6	407,9	0,172	0,067	0,675	0,103	1,920	0,02	331,1	0.24	0,94	0,006	0,007	97,84
B122	27.85	31,30	0,598	0,004	0,057	0.715	0,722	0,01	29,4	1,33	1,07	0,177	0,008	4,08
B127	0,533	0,032	0,067	0,024	0,003	0,063	0,123	0,117	4,27	0.45	0,09	0,347	0,03	0,373
B140	0,106	0,109	0,008	0,0002	0,0006	0,075	0,102	0,032	0,47	0.49	0,05	0,01	0,02	0,841
B15	3,273	3,534	0.18	0,011	0,005	0,176	0,987	0,203	3,52	1.62	0,07	1,75	0,02	0,043
B18	0,495	0,692	0,021	0,062	0,006	0,178	0,214	0,227	1,64	0,13	0,07	0,013	0,04	0,199
B35	0,862	2,959	0,162	0,127	0,004	0,109	0,635	0,161	3,5	0,89	0,06	0,65	3,69	0,127
B43	4,950	1,066	0,685	0,609	0,012	0,410	0,75	2,382	2,48	1.06	0,14	0,023	0,12	6,077
B50	51,18	0,260	1,409	2,02	2,9-5	0,0005	0.99	0,064	2,54	0.81	2,18	0,002	0,26	0,221
B152	4,046	0,550	0.46	0,598	0,0006	1.402	0,107	0,051	0,31	0.28	0,21	0,033	0,41	0,151
B172	3,041	0,373	0,099	0,404	1,7'β	4E-05	0,176	0,01	0,58	0.24	0,04	0,009	0,07	0,35
B175	10,37	0,196	0,494	1,919	2,2-5	0,0003	0,3	0,009	0,39	1,05	0,002	0,011	0,04	0,799
B190	8,037	0,707	0,013	0,035	0,001	1,160	1,334	1,188	0,12	0,01	0,3	0,107	0,57	51,21
B206	10 49	1,641	0,868	0,373	0,0005	0,005	1.02	0,316	0,38	0.42	0,16	0,052	0,23	27,63
B207	0,606	0,146	0,005	0,014	1,2's	0.002	0,383	0,042	5,26	0.21	0,51	0,073	0,3	1,031
B213	0,360	0,543	0,01	0,021	5,7-e	0,000	0,4	0,097	0,08	0,13	0,13	0,128	0,009	0,2
B214	0,238	0,105	0,005	0,017	ı,r5	0.000	0,296	0,387	0,02	0,22	0,02	0,05	0,37	0,096
19	0,922	0,260	0,044	0,198	0,0005	0,537	0,911	1,528	0,04	1,33	0,28	0,132	0,76	0,009

Annex E - Mean relapse-free survival (RFS) and cancer-specific survival (CSS) in months for the 14 miRNAs studied.

cancer-specific survival (CSS) in months for the 14 miRNAs studied

1: cases below average expression; 2: cases above average expression

	SLR pTa (n=30)		SLR pT2/pT3 (n=30)		SCE pT2/pT3 (n=30)	
miRNA		**p**		**p**		**p**
100	21,79 (1) 22,37 (2)	0,45	21,63 (1) 21,67 (2)	0,55	22,6 (1) 26,23 (2)	0,57
10a	22,54 (1) 19,12 (2)	0,83	26,13 (1) 13,05 (2)	**0,007**	27,34 (1) 15,28 (2)	**0,04**
21	24,58 (1) 16,32 (2)	**0,02**	22,4 (1) 13,5 (2)	0,85	25,04 (1) 13,5 (2)	0,49

205	23,82 (1) 19,06 (2)	0,24	21,92 (1) 18 (2)	0,63	21,2 (1) 30,4 (2)	0,08
Let7c	21,39 (1) 27,33 (2)	0,43	21,9 (1) 23,25 (2)	0,96	21,39 (1) 34 (2)	0,12
125b	23,78 (1) 17,44 (2)	0,24	21,5 (1) 23,16 (2)	0,9	21,35 (1) 34 (2)	0,11
143	21,39 (1) 27,33 (2)	0,43	22,2 (1) 15 (2)	0,92	24,88 (1) 15 (2)	0,73
145	22,04 (1) 23,07 (2)	0,95	25,19 (1) 15,57 (2)	**0,03**	24,76 (1) 23,13 (2)	0,62
221	22,86 (1) 21,33 (2)	0,7	21,79 (1) 20,73 (2)	0,68	23,5 (1) 23,85 (2)	0,5
223	22,86 (1) 21,33 (2)	0,7	21,47 (1) 20,61 (2)	0,61	24,5 (1) 22,2 (2)	0,93
15a	22,98 (1) 20,87 (2)	0,66	22,4 (1) 13,5 (2)	0,85	26,57 (1) 18,96 (2)	0,32
16-1	23,55 (1) 17,2 (2)	0,19	23,95 (1) 18,3 (2)	0,5	25,67 (1) 21,99 (2)	0,81
199a	22,19 (1) 22,33 (2)	0,97	22,78 (1) 18,86 (2)	0,69	22,87 (1) 24,8 (2)	0,29
452	23,95 (1) 20,92 (2)	0,37	19,19 (1) 30,8 (2)	0,11	23,77 (1) 27 (2)	0,72

8. BIBLIOGRAPHICAL REFERENCES

Agirre X, Jiménez-Velasco A, San José-Enériz E, , Bandrés E, Garate LCordeu L, Aparicio O, Saez B, Navarro G, Vilas-Zornoza A, Pérez-Roger I, Garcia-Foncillas J, Torres A, Calasanz MJ, Heiniger A, Fortes P, Romàn-Gómez J, Prósper F. Down-regulation of hsa-miR-10a in chronic myeloid leukemia CD34+ cells increases USF2-mediated cell growth. *Mol Cancer Res.* 2008;6(12):1830-40.

Ambros V. MicroRNA Pathways in Flies and Worms: growth, death, fat, stress and timing. *Cell.* 2003;113(6):673-76.

Babjuk M, Oosterlinck W, Sylvester R, Kaasinen E, Bohle A, Palou-Redorta J. EAU Guidelines on Non-Muscle-Carcinoma of the Bladder. *Actas Urol Espn.* 2009;33(4):361-71.

Bakkar AA, Wallerand H, Radvanyi F, Lahaye JB, Pissard S, Lecerf L, Kouyoumdjian JC, Abbou CC, Pairon JC, Jaurand MC, Thiery JP, Chopin DK, de Medina SGD. FGFR3 and TP53 Gene Mutations Define Two Distinct Pathways in Urothelial Cell Carcinoma of Bladder. *Cancer Res.* 2003;63(23):8108-12.

Bartel DP, Chen C. Micromanagers of gene expression: the potentially widespread influence of metazoan microRNAs. *Nat Rev Genet.* 2004;5:396-400.

Bartel DP. MicroRNAs: Genomics, Biogenesis, Mechanism, and Function. *Cell.* 2004;116(2):281-297.

Belakhlef S, Church C, Jani C, Lakhanpal S. Early Dynamic PET/CT and 18F-FDG Blood Flow Imaging in Bladder Cancer Detection: A Novel Approach. *Clin Nucl Med.* 2012;37(4):366-8.

Bessière D, Lacroix C, Campagne S, Ecochard V, Guillet V, Mourey L, Lopez F, Czaplicki J, Demange P, Milon A, Girard JP, Gervais V. Structure-function analysis of the THAP zinc finger of THAP1, a large C2CH DNA-binding module linked to Rb/E2F pathways. *J Biol Chem*. 2008;283(7):4352-63.

Blenkiron C, Miska E. MiRNAs in cancer: approaches, aetiology, diagnostics and therapy. *Hum Mol Genet*. 2007;16:106-13.

Boffetta P, Silverman DT. A meta-analysis of bladder cancer and diesel exhaust exposure. *Epidemiology*. 2001 ;12(1):125-30.

Borden LS, Clark PE, Hall MC. Bladder Cancer. *Curr Opin Oncol*. 2005;17(3):275-80.

Botteman MF, Pashos CL, Radaelli A, Laskin B, Hauser R. The health economics of bladder cancer: a comprehensive review of the published literature. *Pharmacoeconomics*. 2003;21:1315-30.

Bozhenok L, Wade PA, Varga-Weisz P. WSTF-ISWI chromatin remodeling complex targets heterochromatic replication foci. *EMBO J*. 2002;21(9):2231-41.

Brabletz S, Brabletz T. The ZEB/miR-200 feedback loop - a motor of cellular plasticity in development and cancer? *EMBO Reports*. 2010;11(9):670-77.

Brait M, Begum S, Carvalho AL, Dasgupta S, Vettore AL, Czerniak B, Caballero OL, Westra WH, Sidransky D, Hoque MO. Aberrant promoter methylation of multiple genes during pathogenesis of bladder cancer. *Cancer Epidemiol Biomarkers Prev*. 2008;17(10):2786-94.

Calin GA, Croce CM. MicroRNA signatures in human cancers. *Nat Rev Cancer*. 2006;6(11):857-66.

Calin GA, Dumitru CD, Shimizu M, Bichi R, Zupo S, Noch E, Aldler H, Rattan S, Keating M, Rai K, Rassenti L, Kipps T, Negrini M, Bullrich F, Croce CM. Frequent deletions and down-regulation of micro- RNA genes miR15 and miR16 at 13q14 in chronic lymphocytic leukemia. *PNAS*. 2002;99(24):15524-9.

Cantor KP, Lynch CF, Johnson D. Bladder cancer, parity, and age at first birth.

Cancer Causes Control. 1992;3(1):57-62.

Cappellen D, Oliveira C, Ricol D, Medina SGD. Frequent activating mutations of FGFR3 in human bladder and cervix carcinomas. *Nat Genet*. 1999;23:18-20.

Carmell MA, Hannon GJ. RNase III enzymes and the initiation of gene silencing. *Nat Struct Mol Biol*. 2004;11(3):214-8.

Catto JWF, Miah S, Owen HC, Bryant H, Myers K, Dudziec E, Larré S, Milo M, Rehman I, Rosario DJ, Di Martino E, Knowles MA, Meuth M, Harris AL, Hamdy FC. Distinct microRNA alterations characterize high and low grade bladder cancer. *Cancer Res*. 2009;69(21):8472-81.

Chen R, Alvero AB, Silasi DA, Kelly MG, Fest S, Visintin I, Leiser A, Schwartz PE, Rutherford T, Mor G. Regulation of IKKbeta by miR-199a affects NF-kappaB activity in ovarian cancer cells. *Oncogene*. 2008;27(34):4712-23.

Chen X, Ba Y, Ma L, Cai X, Yin Y, Wang K, Guo J, Zhang Y, Chen J, Guo X, Li Q, Li X, Wang J, Jiang X, Xiang Y, Xu C, Zheng P, Li R, Zhang H, Shang X, Gong T, Ning G, Wang J, Zen K, Zhang J, Zhang C. characterization of microRNAs in serum: a novel class of biomarkers for diagnosis of cancer and other diseases. *Cell Res*. 2008;18:997-1006.

Cheung HH, Davis AJ, Lee TL, Pang AL, Nagrani S, Rennert OM, Chan WY. Methylation of an intronic region regulates miR-199a in testicular tumor malignancy. *Oncogene*. 2011;30(31):3404-15

Chiyomaru T, Enokida H, Tatarano S, Kawahara K, Uchida Y, Nishiyama K, Fujimura L, Kikkawa N, Seki N, Nakagawa M. miR-145 and miR-133a function as tumor suppressors and directly regulate FSCN1 expression in bladder cancer. *British J Cancer*. 2010;102(5):883-891.

Cimmino A, Calin GA, Fabbri M, Iorio MV, Ferracin M, Shimizu M, Wojcik SE, Aqeilan R, Zupo S, Dono M, Rassenti L, Alder H, Volinia S, Liu C, Kipps TJ, Negrini M, Croce CM. miR-15 and miR-16 induce apoptosis by targeting BCL2.

PNAS. 2005;102(39):13944-49.

Cordon-Cardo C, Wartinger D, Petrylak D, Dalbagni G, Fair WR, Fuks Z, Reuter VE. Altered expression of the retinoblastoma gene product: prognostic indicator in bladder cancer. *J Natl Cancer Inst*. 1992;84(16):1251-6.

Dalmay T. MicroRNAs and cancer. *J Intern Med*. 2008;263(4):366-75.

Der CJ, Krontiris TG, Cooper GM. Transforming genes of human bladder and lung carcinoma cell lines are homologous to the ras genes of Harvey and Kirsten sarcoma viruses. *PNAS*. 1982;79(11):3637-40.

Desai S, Lim SD, Jimenez RE, Chun T, Keane TE, McKenney JK, Zavala-Pompa A, Cohen C, Young RH, Amin MB. Relationship of cytokeratin 20 and CD44 protein expression with WHO/ISUP grade in pTa and pT1 papillary urothelial neoplasia. *Mod Pathol*. 2000;13(12):1315-23.

Dip N, Reis ST, Timoszczuk LS, Abe, DK, DallOglio M, Srougi M, Leite KRM. Under-expression of miR-100 may be a new carcinogenic pathway for low grade pTa bladder urothelial carcinomas. *Mol Biomark Diagn*. 2011;2(6):2-6.

Duan Z, Choy E, Harmon D, Liu X, Susa M, Mankin H, Hornicek F. MicroRNA-199a-3p is downregulated in human osteosarcoma and regulates cell proliferation and migration. *Mol Cancer Ther*. 2011;10(8):1337-45.

Eisner BH, Feldman AS. Nanoparticle imaging for genitourinary cancers. *Cancer Biomarkers*. 2009;5:75-9.

Ellinger J, El Kassem N, Heukamp LC, Matthews S, Cubukluoz F, Kahl P, Perabo FG, Müller SC, von Ruecker A, Bastian PJ. Hypermethylation of cell-free serum DNA indicates worse outcome in patients with bladder cancer. *J Urol*. 2008;179(1):346-52.

Enokida H, Nakagawa M. Epigenetics in bladder cancer. *Int J Clin Oncol*. 2008;13(4):298-307.

Esrig D, Elmajian D, Groshen S, Freeman JA, Stein JP, Chen SC, Nichols PW,

Skinner DG, Jones PA, Cote RJ. Accumulation of nuclear p53 and tumor progression in bladder cancer. *N Engl J Med.* 1994;331(19):1259-64.

Foley NH, Bray I, Watters KM, Das S, Bryan K, Bernas T, Prehn JH, Stallings RL. MicroRNAs 10a and 10b are potent inducers of neuroblastoma cell differentiation through targeting of nuclear receptor corepressor 2. *Cell Death Differ.* 2011;18(7):1089-98.

Fornari F, Milazzo M, Chieco P, Negrini M, Calin GA, Grazi GL, Pollutri D, Croce CM, Bolondi L, Gramantieri L. MiR-199a-3p regulates mTOR and c-Met to influence the doxorubicin sensitivity of human hepatocarcinoma cells. *Cancer Res.* 2010;70(12):5184-93.

Friedrich MG, Chandrasoma S, Siegmund KD, Weisenberger DJ, Cheng JC, Toma MI, Huland H, Jones PA, Liang G. Prognostic relevance of methylation markers in patients with non-muscle invasive bladder carcinoma. *Eur J Cancer.* 2005;41(17):2769-78.

Fritsche HM, Burger M, Svatek RS, Jeldres C, Karakiewicz PI, Novara G, Skinner E, Denzinger S, Fradet Y, Isbarn H, Bastian PJ, Volkmer BG, Montorsi F, Kassouf W, Tilki D, Otto W, Capitanio U, Izawa JI, Ficarra V, Lerner S, Sagalowsky AI, Schoenberg M, Kamat A, Dinney CP, Lotan Y, Shariat SF. Characteristics and outcomes of patients with clinical T1 grade 3 urothelial carcinoma treated with radical cystectomy: results from an international cohort. *Eur Urol.* 2010;57(2):300-9.

Gaertner RR, Thériault GP. Risk of bladder cancer in foundry workers: a metaanalysis. *Occup Environ Med.* 2002;59(10):655-63.

Gallucci M, Guadagni F, Marzano R, Leonardo C, Merola R, Sentinelli S, Ruggeri EM, Cantiani R, Sperduti I, Lopez Fde L, Cianciulli AM. Status of the p53, p16, RB1, and HER-2 genes and chromosomes 3, 7, 9, and 17 in advanced bladder cancer: correlation with adjacent mucosa and pathological parameters. *J Clin Pathol.* 2005;58(4):367-71.

Gandellini P, Folini M, Longoni N, Pennati M, Binda M, Colecchia M, Salvioni R, Supino R, Moretti RValdagni R, Limonta P, , Daidone MG, Zaffaroni N. miR-205 Exerts tumor-suppressive functions in human prostate through downregulation of protein kinase Cepsilon. *Cancer Res.* 2009;69(6):2287-95.

Garcia del Muro X, Condom E, Vigués F, Castellsagué X, Figueras A, Munoz J, Solà J, Soler T, Capellà G, Germà JR. p53 and p21 Expression levels predict organ preservation and survival in invasive bladder carcinoma treated with a combined-modality approach. *Cancer.* 2004;100(9):1859-67.

Garzon R, Pichiorri F, Palumbo T, Iuliano R, Cimmino A, Aqeilan R, Volinia S, Bhatt D, Alder H, Marcucci G, Calin GA, Liu C, Bloomfield CD, Andreeff M, Croce CM. MicroRNA fingerprints during human megakaryocytopoiesis. *PNAS.* 2006;106(13):5078-83.

Gore JL, Lai J, Setodji CM, Litwin MS, Saigal CS; Urologic Diseases in America Project. Mortality increases when radical cystectomy is delayed more than 12 weeks: results from a Surveillance, Epidemiology, and End Results-Medicare analysis. *Cancer.* 2009;115(5):988-96.

Gottardo F, Liu CG, Ferracin M, Calin GA, Fassan M, Bassi P, Sevignani C, Byrne D, Negrini M, Pagano F, Gomella LG, Croce CM, Baffa R. Micro-RNA profiling in kidney and bladder cancers. *Urol Oncol.* 2007;25(5):387-92.

Gregory RI, Yan K, Amuthan G, Chendrimada TP, Doratotaj B, Cooch N, Shiekhattar R. The Microprocessor complex mediates the genesis of microRNAs. *Nature.* 2004;432:235-240.

Gregory PA, Bert AG, Paterson EL, Barry SC, Tsykin A, Farshid G, Vadas MA, Khew-Goodall Y, Goodall GJ. The miR-200 family and miR-205 regulate epithelial to mesenchymal transition by targeting ZEB1 and SIP1. *Nat Cell Biol.* 2008;10(5):593-601.

Guan Y, Yao H, Zheng Z, Qiu G, Sun K. MiR-125b targets BCL3 and suppresses ovarian cancer proliferation. *Int J Cancer.* 2011;128(10):2274-83.

Hainaut P, Hollstein M. p53 and human cancer: the first ten thousand mutations. *Adv Cancer* Res. 2000;77:81-137.

Han J, Lee Y, Yeom KH, Kim YK, Jin H, Kim VN. The Drosha-DGCR8 complex in primary microRNA processing. *Genes Dev*. 2004;18(24):3016-27.

Heney NM. Natural history of superficial bladder cancer. Prognostic features and long-term disease course. *Urol Clin North Am*. 1992;19(3):429-33.

Henson BJ, Bhattacharjee S, O'Dee DM, Feingold E, Gollin SM. Decreased expression of miR-125b and miR-100 in oral cancer cells contributes to malignancy. *Genes Chromosomes Cancer*. 2009;48(7):569-82.

Herr H, Lee C, Chang S, Lerner S. Standardization of radical cystectomy and pelvic lymph node dissection for bladder cancer: a collaborative group report. *J Urol*. 2004;171(5):1823-8.

Huang L, Luo J, Cai Q, Pan Q, Zeng H, Guo Z, Dong W, Huang J, Lin T. MicroRNA-125b suppresses the development of bladder cancer by targeting E2F3. *Int J Cancer*. 2011;128(8):1758-69.

Huang H, Xie C, Sun X, Ritchie RP, Zhang J, Chen YE. miR-10a contributes to retinoid acid-induced smooth muscle cell differentiation. *J Biol Chem*. 2010;285(13):9383-9.

Ichimi T, Enokida H, Okuno Y, Kunimoto R, Chiyomaru T, Kawamoto K, Kawahara K, Toki K, Kawakami K, Nishiyama K, Tsujimoto G, Nakagawa M, Seki N. Identification of novel microRNA targets based on microRNA signatures in bladder cancer. *Int J Cancer*. 2009;125:345-52.

INCA (National Cancer Institute) [on-line]. Ministry of Health, Brazil; 2011. Available from: http://www.inca.gov.br.

Izzoti A, Calin GA, Arrigo P, Steele VE, Croce CM, De Flora S. Downregulation of microRNA expression in the lungs of rats exposed to cigarette smoke. *Faseb J*. 2009; 23(3);806-12.

Jebar AH, Hurst CD, Tomlinson DC, Johnston C, Taylor CF, Knowles MA. FGFR3 and Ras gene mutations are mutually exclusive genetic events in urothelial cell carcinoma. *Oncogene*. 2005;24:5218-25.

Jemal A, Bray F, Center MM, Ferlay Ward E, Forman D. Global Cancer Statistics, 2011. *Cancer J Clin*. 2011;61(2):69-90.

Johnson SM, Grosshans H, Shingara J, Byrom M, Jarvis R, Cheng A, Labourier E, Reinert KL, Brown D, Slack FJ. RAS is Regulated by the let-7 MicroRNA Family. *Cell*. 2005;120(5):635-47.

Kim YT, Park SJ, Lee SH, Kang HJ, Hahn S, Kang CH, Sung SW, Kim JH. Prognostic implication of aberrant promoter hypermethylation of CpG islands in adenocarcinoma of the lung. *J Thorac Cardiovasc Surg*. 2005;130(5):1378.

Kim VN. MicroRNA Biogenesis: Coordinated Cropping and Dicing. *Nature*. 2005;6:376-385.

Kirkali Z, Chan T, Manoharan M, Algaba F, Busch C, Cheng L, Kiemeney L, Kriegmair M, Montironi R, Murphy WM, Sesterhenn IA, Tachibana M, Weider J. Bladder Cancer: Epidemiology, Staging and Grading, and Diagnosis. *Urology*. 2005;66(6):4-34.

Klussmann JH, Li Z, Bohmer K, Maroz A, Koch ML, Emmrich S, Godinho FJ, Orkin SH, Reinhardt D. miR-125b-2 is a potential oncomiR on human chromosome 21 in megakaryoblastic leukemia. *Gen Dev*. 2010;24(5):478-90.

Knowles MA. Molecular pathogenesis of bladder cancer. *Int J Clin Oncol*. 2008;13(4):287-97.

Laios A, O'Toole S, Flavin R, Martin C, Kelly L, Ring M, Finn SP, Barrett C, Loda M, Gleeson N, D'Arcy T, McGuinness E, Sheils O, Sheppard B, O'Leary J. Potential role of mir-9 and mir-223 in recurrent ovarian cancer. *Mol Cancer*. 2008;7:35.

Le MTN, Teh C, Shyh-Chang N, Xie H, Zhou B, Korzh V, Lodish HE, Lim B. MicroRNA-125b is a novel negative regulator of p53. *Gene Dev*. 2009;23:1-15.

Lebanony D, Benjamin H, Gilad S, Ezagouri M, Dov A, Ashkenazi K, Gefen N, Izraeli S, Rechavi G, Pass H, Nonaka D, Li J, Spector Y, Rosenfeld N, Chajut A, Cohen D, Aharonov R, Mansukhani M. Diagnostic assay based on hsa-miR-205 expression distinguishes squamous from nonsquamous non-small-cell lung carcinoma. *J Clin Oncol.* 2009;27(12):2030-37.

Lee RC, Feinbaum RL, Ambros V. The *C. elegans* Heterochronic Gene lin-4 Encodes Small RNAs with Antisense Complementarity to lin-14. *Cell.* 1993;75:843-854.

Lee Y, Ahn C, Han J, Chol H, Kim J, Yim J, Lee J, Provost P, Radmark O, Kim S, Kim VN. The nuclear Rnase III Drosha initiates microRNA processing. *Nature.* 2003;425:415-418.

Lee YS, Nakahara K, Pham JW, Kim K, He Z, Sontheimer EJ, Carthew RW. Disctinct Roles for *Drosophila* Dicer-1 and Dicer-2 in the siRNA/miRNA Silencing Pathways. *Cell.* 2004;117:69-81.

Leite KRM, Sousa-Canavez JM, Reis ST, Tomiyama A, Camara-Lopes LH, Sanudo A, Antunes AA, Srougi M. Change in expression of miR-let7c, miR-100, and miR-218 from high grade localized prostate cancer to metastasis. *Urol Oncol.* 2009;29(3):265-269.

Lewis BP, Burge CB, Bartel DP. Conserved Seed Pairing, Often Flanked by Adenosines, Indicates that Thousands of Human Genes are MicroRNA Targets. *Cell.* 2005;120(1):15-20.

Liang L, Wong C, Ying Q, Fan DY, Huang S, Ding J, Yao J, Yan M, Li J, Yao M, Ng IO, He X. MicroRNA-125b Suppressed Human Liver Cancer Cell Proliferation and Metastasis by Directly Targeting Oncogene LIN28B. Hepatology. 2010;52(5):1731-40.

Lin T, Dong W, Huang J, Pan Q, Fan X, Zhang C, Huang L. MicroRNA-143 as a Tumor Suppressor for Bladder Cancer. *J Urol.* 2009;181(3):1372-80.

Lodygin D, Tarasov V, Epanchintsev A, Berking C, Knyazeva T, Korner H,

Knyazev P, Diebold J, Hermeking H. Inactivation of miR-34a by aberrant CpG methylation in multiple types of cancer. *Cell Cycle*. 2008;7(16):2591-600.

Lu Q, Lu C, Zhou G, Zhang WZ, Xiao H, Wang X. MicroRNA-221 silencing predisposed human bladder cancer cells to undergo apoptosis induced by TRAIL. *Urol Oncol*. 2010;28:635-41.

Ma L, Teruya-Feldstein J, Weinberg RA. Tumor invasion and metastasis initiated by microRNA-10b in breast cancer. *Nature*. 2007;449(7163):682-88.

Markowitz SB, Levin K. Continued Epidemic of Bladder Cancer in Workers Exposed to Ortho-Toluidine in a Chemical Factory. J Occup Environ Med 2004;46(2):154-60.

Marsit CJ, Houseman EA, Schned AR, Karagas MR, Kelsey KT. Promoter hypermethylation is associated with current smoking, age, gender and survival in bladder cancer. *Carcinogenesis*. 2007;28(8):1745-51.

Martinez-Torrecuadrada J, Cifuentes G, López-Serra P, Saenz P, Martinez A, Casal JI. Targeting the Extracellular Domain of Fibroblast Growth Factor Receptor 3 with Human Single-Chain Fv Antibodies Inhibits Bladder Carcinoma Cell Line Proliferation. *Clin Cancer Res*. 2005;11(17):6280-90.

Mascaux C, Laes JF, Anthoine G, Haller A, Ninane V, Burny A, Sculier JP. Evolution of microRNA expression during human bronchial squamous carcinogenesis. *Eur Respir J*. 2009;33(2):352-9.

McConkey DJ, Lee S, Choi W, Tran M, Majewski T, Lee S, Siefker-Radtke A, Dinney C, Czerniak B. Molecular genetics of bladder cancer: Emerging mechanisms of tumor initiation and progression. *Urol Oncol*. 2010;28(4):429-40.

Meister G, Landthaler M, Patkaniowska A, Dorsett Y, Tuschl T. Sequencespecific inhibition of microRNA- and siRNA-induced RNA silencing. *RNA*. 2004;10:544-550.

Meng F, Henson R, Wehbe-Janek H, Ghoshal K, Jacob ST, Patel T.

MicroRNA-21 Regulates Expression of the PTEN Tumor Suppressor Gene in Human Hepatocellular Cancer. *Gastroenterology*. 2007;133:647-58.

Miyamoto H, Epstein JI. Transurethral resection specimens of the bladder: outcome of invasive urothelial cancer involving muscle bundles indeterminate between muscularis mucosae and muscularis propria. *Urology*. 2010;76(3):600-2.

Mo L, Zheng X, Huang HY, Shapiro E, Lepor H, Cordon-Cardo C, Sun TT, Wu XR. Hyperactivation of Ha-ras oncogene, but not Ink4a/Arf deficiency, triggers bladder tumorigenesis. *J Clin Invest*. 2007;117(2):314-25.

Montie JE, Clark PE, Eisenberger MA, El-Galley R, Greenberg RE, Herr HW, Hudes GR, Kuban DA, Kuzel TM, Lange PH, Lele SM, Michalski J, Patterson A, Pohar KS, Richie JP, Sexton WJ, Shipley WU, Small EJ, Trump DL, Walther PJ, Wilson TG. Bladder cancer. *J Natl Compr Canc Netw*. 2009;7(1):8-39.

Mungan NA, Aben KK, Schoenberg MP, Visser O, Coebergh JW, Witjes JA, Kiemeney LA. Gender differences in stage-adjusted bladder cancer survival. *Urology*. 2000;55(6):876-80.

Nagaraja AK, Creighton CJ, Yu Z, Zhu H, Gunaratne PH, Reid JG, Olokpa E, Itamochi H, Ueno NT, Hawkins SM, Anderson ML, Matzuk MM. A link between miR-100 and FRAP1/mTOR in clear cell ovarian cancer. *Mol Endocrinol*. 2010;24(2):447-63.

Neely LA, Rieger-Christ KM, Neto BS, Eroshkin A, Garver J, Patel S, Phung NA, McLaughlin S, Libertino JA, Whitney D, Summerhayes IC. A microRNA expression ratio defining the invasive phenotype in bladder tumors. *Urol Oncol*. 2008;28(1):39-48.

Ornitz DM, Xu J, Colvin JS, McEwen DG, MacArthur CA, Coulier F, Gao G, Goldfarb M. Receptor Specificity of the Fibroblast Growth Factor Family. *Journal Biol Chem*. 1996;271(25):15292-97.

Orom UA, Nielsen FC, Lund AH. microRNA-10a binds the 5'UTR of ribosomal protein mRNA and enhances their translation. *Mol Cell*. 2008;30(4):460-71.

Ozen M, Creighton CJ, Ozdemir M, Ittmann M. Widespread deregulation of microRNA expression in human prostate cancer. *Oncogene*. 2008;27(12):1788-93.

Paik ML, Scolieri MJ, Brown SL, Spirnak JP, Resnick MI. Limitations of Computerized Tomography in Staging Invasive Bladder Cancer before Radical Cystectomy. *J Urol*. 2000;163:1693-96.

Pandith AA, Shah ZA, Siddiqi MA. Oncogenic role of fibroblastic growth factor receptor 3 in tumorigenesis of urinary bladder cancer. *Urol Oncol*. 2010 (Epub ahead of print).

Pillai RS, Bhattacharyya SN, Artus CG, Zoller T, Cougot N, Basyuk E, E, Bertrand Filipowicz W. Inhibition of translational initiation by Let-7 MicroRNA in human cells. *Science*. 2005;309(5740):1573-6.

Pillai, RS. MicroRNA function: Multiple mechanisms for a tiny RNA? *RNA*. 2005;11:1753-1761.

Pineau P, Volinia S, McJunkin K, Marchio A, Battiston C, Terris B, Mazzaferro V, Lowe SW, Croce CM, Dejean A. miR-221 overexpression contributes to liver tumorigenesis. *PNAS*. 2010;107(1):264-9.

Proctor I, Stoeber K, Williams GH. Biomarkers in bladder cancer. *Histopathology*. 2010;57:1-13.

Przybojewska B, Jagiello A, Jalmuzna P. H-RAS, K-RAS, and N-RAS gene activation in human bladder cancers. *Cancer Genet Cytogenet*. 2000;121(1):73-7.

PubMed - US National Library of Medicine - National Institutes of Health; 2012 Available from: http://www.ncbi.nlm.nih.gov/sites/entrez.

Puzio-Kuter AM, Castillo-Martin M, Kinkade CW, Wang X, Shen TH, Matos T, Shen MM, Cordon-Cardo C, Abate-Shen C. Inactivation of p53 and Pten promotes invasive bladder cancer. *Gene Dev.* 2009;23:675-80.

Rajabi H, Jin C, Ahmad R, McClary AC, Joshi MD, Kufe D. Mucin I Oncoprotein Expression Is Suppressed by the miR-125b Oncomir. *Genes and Cancer.* 2010;1(1):62-68.

Reinhart BJ, Slack FJ, Basson M, Pasquinelli AE, Bettinger JC, Rougvle AE, Horvitz HR, Ruvkun G. The 21-nucleotide let-7 RNA regulates developmental timing in Caenorhabditis elegans. *Nature.* 2000;403:901-906.

Rieger-Christ KM, Mourtzinos A, Lee PJ, Zagha RM, Cain J, Silverman M, Libertino JA, Summerhayes IC. Identification of fibroblast growth factor receptor 3 mutations in urine sediment DNA samples complements cytology in bladder tumor detection. *Cancer.* 2003;98(4):737-44.

Sachdeva M, Mo Y. MiR-145 Suppresses Cell Invasion and Metastasis by Directly Targeting Mucin 1. *Cancer Res.* 2010;70(1):378-387.

Sachdeva M, Mo Y. miR-145-mediated suppression of cell growth, invasion and metastasis. *Am J Transl Res.* 2010;2(2):170-180.

Sachdeva M, Zhu S, Wu F, Wu H, Walia V, Kumar S, Elble R, Watabe K, Mo YY. p53 reppresses c-Myc through induction of the tumor suppressor miR-145. *PNAS.* 2009;106(9): 3207-12.

Sage C, Nagel R, Egan DA, Schrier M, Mesman E, Mangiola A, Anile C, Maira G, Mercatelli N, Ciafrè SA, Farace MG, Agami R. Regulation of the p27kip1 tumor suppressor by miR-221 and miR-222 promotes cancer cell proliferation. *EMBO J.* 2007;26:3699-3708.

Sarkis AS, Dalbagni G, Cordon-Cardo C, Melamed J, Zhang ZF, Sheinfeld J, Fair WR, Herr HW, Reuter VE. Association of P53 nuclear overexpression and tumor progression in carcinoma in situ of the bladder. *J Urol.* 1994;152(2 Pt 1):388-92.

Shi X, Xue L, Ma A, Tepper CG, Kung HJ, White Wd. miR-12b Promotes Growth of Prostate Cancer Xenograft Tumor through Targeting Pro-Apoptotic

Genes. *The Prostate*. 2011;71:538-49.

Si ML, Zhu S, Wu H, Lu Z, Wu F, Mo YY. miR-21-mediated tumor growth. *Oncogene*. 2006;1-5.

Spizzo R, Nicoloso MS, Lupini L, Lu Y, Fogarty J, Rossi S, Zagatti B, Fabbri M, Veronese A, Liu X, Davuluri R, Croce CM, Mills G, Negrini M, Calin GA. miR- 145 participates with TP53 in death-promoting regulatory loop and targets estrogen receptor-α in human breast cancer cells. *Cell Death and Differentiation*. 2010; 17(2): 246-54.

Stamatopoulos B, Meuleman N, Haibe-Kains B, Saussoy P, Neste EVD, Michaux L, Heimann P, Martiat P, Bron D, Lagneaux L. microRNA-29c and microRNA-223 down-regulation has in vivo significance in chronic lymphocytic leukemia and improves disease risk stratification. *Blood*. 2009;113(21):5237-45.

Suzuki HI, Yamagata K, Sugimoto K, Iwamoto T, Kato S, Miyazono K. Modulation of microRNA processing by p53. *Nature*. 2009;460:529-34.

The miRNA body map; 2011. Available from:

http://www.mirnabodymap.org/mirna_card.php.

Thériault G, Tremblay C, Cordier S, Gingras S. Bladder cancer in the aluminium industry. *Lancet*. 1984;1(8383):947-50.

Thompson LM, Plummer S, Schalling M, Altherr MR, Gusella JF, Housman DE, Wasmuth JJ. A gene encoding a fibroblast growth factor receptor isolated from the Huntington disease gene region of human chromosome 4. *Genomics*. 1991;11(4):1133-42.

Tomlinson DC, Baldo O, Harnden P, Knowles MA. FGFR3 protein expression and its relationship to mutation status and prognostic variables in bladder cancer. *J Pathol*. 2007;213(1):91-98.

Tritchler S, Mosler C, Straub J, Buchner A, Karl A, Graser A, Stief C, Tilki D.

Staging of muscle-invasive bladder cancer: can computerized tomography help us to decide on local treatment? *World J Urol.* 2011 (Epub ahead of print).

Tsuruta H, Kishimoto H, Sasaki T, Horie Y, Natsui M, Shibata Y, Hamada KKawahara K, Yajima N, , Sasaki M, Tsuchiya N, Enomoto K, Mak TW, Nakano T, Habuchi T, Suzuki A. Hyperplasia and carcinomas in Pten-deficient mice and reduced PTEN protein in human bladder cancer patients. *Cancer Res.* 2006;66(17):8389-96.

van der Weyden L, Adams DJ. The Ras-association domain family (RASSF) members and their role in human tumourigenesis. *Biochim Biophys Acta.* 2007;1776(1):58

van Rhijn BW, Lurkin I, Radvanyi F, Kirkels WJ, van der Kwast TH, Zwarthoff EC. The Fibroblast Growth Factor Receptor 3 (*FGFR3*) Mutation Is a Strong Indicator of Superficial Bladder Cancer with Low Recurrence Rate. *Cancer Res.* 2001;61:1265-68.

van Rhijn BWG, van der Kwast TH, Vis AN, Kirkels WJ, Boevé ER, Jobsis AC, Zwarthoff EC. FGFR3 and P53 Characterize Alternative Genetic Pathways in the Pathogenesis of Urothelial Cell Carcinoma. *Cancer Res.* 2004;64(6):1911-14.

Veerla S, Lindgren D, Kvist A, Frigyesi A, Staaf J, Persson H, Liedberg F, Chebil G, Gudjonsson S, Borg A, Mansson W, Rovira C, Hoglund M. MiRNA expression in urothelial carcinomas: important roles of miR-10a, miR-222, miR-125b, miR-7 and miR-452 for tumor stage and metastasis, and frequent homozygous losses of miR-31. *Int J Cancer.* 2009;124(9):2236-42.

Weiss FU, Marques IJ, Woltering JM, Vlecken DH, Aghdassi A, Partecke LI, Heidecke CD, Lerch MM, Bagowski CP. Retinoic acid receptor antagonists inhibit miR-10a expression and block metastatic behavior of pancreatic cancer. *Gastroenterology.* 2009;137(6):2136-45.e1-7.

Wiklund ED, Bramsen JB, Hulf T, Dyrskj0t L, Ramanathan R, Hansen TB,

Villadsen SB, Gao S, Ostenfeld MS, Borre M, Peter ME, 0rntoft TF, Kjems J, Clark SJ. Coordinated epigenetic repression of the miR-200 family and miR-205 in invasive bladder cancer. *Int J Cancer*. 2011;128(6):1327-34.

Wong QW, Lung RW, Law PT, Lai PB, Chan KY, To KT, Wong N. MicroRNA-223 Is Commonly Repressed in Hepatocellular Carcinoma and Potentiates Expression of Stathmin1. *Gastroenterology*. 2008;135:257-69.

Wu X. Urothelial Tumorigenesis: A Tale of Divergent Pathways. Nat Rev Cancer 2005;5(9):713-25.

Wu H, Zhu S, Mo Y. Suppression of cell growth and invasion by miR-205 in breast cancer. *Cell Res*. 2009;19:439-48.

Wu XR. Biology of urothelial tumorigenesis: insights from genetically engineered mice. *Cancer Metastasis Rev*. 2009;28(3-4):281-90.

Yates DR, Rehman I, Abbod MF, Meuth M, Cross SS, Linkens DA, Hamdy FC, Catto JW. Promoter hypermethylation identifies progression risk in bladder cancer. Clin *Cancer Res*. 2007;13(7):2046-53.

Yi R, Qin Y, Macara IG, Cullen BR. Exportin-5 mediates the nuclear export of pre-microRNAs and short hairpin RNAs. *Genes Dev*. 2003;17:3011-3016.

Zhou Y, Santoro R, Grummt I. The chromatin remodeling complex NoRC targets HDAC1 to the ribosomal gene promoter and represses RNA polymerase I transcription. *EMBO J*. 2002;21(17):4632-40.

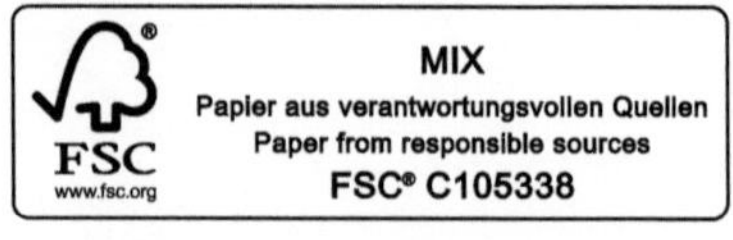

Printed by Books on Demand GmbH, Norderstedt / Germany